From Novice to Expert
*Excellence and Power
in Clinical Nursing Practice*

HE COULD NOT SPEAK, as he was intubated. He could not write, as he was quadriplegic, and we didn't allow him to nod his head due to his unstable neck fracture. His only communication was with his eyes and his amazing ability to mouth words clearly and understandably. . . . I just *knew* we could resolve his problem. . ., so I intervened in his behalf with his multiple physicians. . . . This incident is critical to me because it was what nursing is all about for me. The point was made by one simple statement he mouthed to me later in the day. His words were: "Thank you. You've really helped me a lot. I don't want to imagine what would have happened to me if you weren't here and hadn't cared."

See Chapter 4, "The Helping Role"

"One of the most significant contributions to nursing's literature—for practice, teaching, and theory development."

Rozella Schlotfeldt

"You have demonstrated a way of identifying expertness, and I for one am most grateful to you . . . reading *From Novice to Expert* gave me great pleasure and satisfaction. I hope it will have the greatest possible audience here and abroad."

Virginia Henderson

"The single most data-based work in nursing which deals with practice as a process of striving for excellence. It is a superb work."

Ingeborg G. Mauksch

From Novice to Expert

Excellence and Power in Clinical Nursing Practice

Commemorative Edition

Patricia Benner, R.N., Ph.D.
University of California
School of Nursing
Department of Physiological Nursing

Prentice Hall Health
Upper Saddle River, New Jersey 07458

Library of Congress Cataloging-in-Publication Data
Benner, Patricia E.
   From novice to expert: excellence and power in clinical nursing practice /
Patricia Benner.—Commemorative ed.
        p. cm.
   Prev. published: Menlo Park, Calif.: Addison-Wesley Pub. co.,
   c1984.
   Includes bibliographical references and index.
   ISBN 0-13-032522-8 (pbk.)
   1. Nursing--Practice. 2. Success. I. Title.

   RT82 .B456 2001
   601.73—dc21

                                                              00-059834

Publisher: Julie Alexander
Executive Editor: Maura Connor
Acquisitions Editor: Nancy Anselment
Director of Production and Manufacturing: Bruce Johnson
Managing Editor: Patrick Walsh
Production Editor: Danielle Newhouse
Manufacturing Manager: Ilene Sanford
Creative Director: Marianne Frasco
Printing and Binding: LSC Communications Crawfordsville

Prentice-Hall International (UK) Limited, *London*
Prentice-Hall of Australia Pty. Limited, *Sydney*
Prentice-Hall Canada Inc., *Toronto*
Prentice-Hall Hispanoamericana, S.A., *Mexico*
Prentice-Hall of India Private Limited, *New Delhi*
Prentice-Hall of Japan, Inc., *Tokyo*
Prentice-Hall Singapore Pte. Ltd.
Editora Prentice-Hall do Brasil, Ltda., *Rio de Janeiro*

                                                    26   17
                              ISBN 0-13-032522-8

| Foreword

Prentice-Hall presents this commemorative edition of *From Novice to Expert: Excellence and Power in Clinical Nursing Practice* after sixteen years, ten translations, and a reception to this book that has been extremely gratifying. The goals of the work were to study experiential learning in nursing practice, examine skill acquisition based on clinical learning, and articulate knowledge embedded in nursing practice. Narratives of experiential learning link the learner, context, relationships, and timing. Experience-based narratives tap into common human predicaments and vulnerabilities that may show up differently in other cultural and organizational settings. Readers comment that this work 'puts into words what they have always known but not been able to express about nursing practice'—a perfect compliment since this work seeks to give public, accessible language to a hidden or marginalized practice (i.e., articulation research). Readers are able to compare and contrast similarities and differences between the narratives and their own practical and cultural contexts.

When this work was first published, nurses were beginning to seek long-term careers in clinical practice and were interested in ways of finding development and advancement based on clinical expertise and education. Career advancement had been tied to leaving direct patient care for teaching or administrative work. This work showed why practicing nurse clinicians needed to be retained and rewarded for their clinical expertise in practice settings. This research demonstrates that practice is a way of knowing in its own right. It offers an alternative view of skilled nursing know-how, ongoing clinical inquiry, and the development of clinical knowledge in nursing practice. As a member-participant in nursing's tradition of practice, each nurse stands on the shoulders of past and present colleagues. How we treat our daily experiential learning in clinical practice determines the extent to which our research and education will become both collective and cumulative, and vitally connected to clinical practice.

Nursing as a practice–a socially organized and embedded form of knowledge and ethics–like any practice continually faces challenges of development or decline. Practices grow through experiential learning and through transmitting that learning in practical settings. Practices cannot be completely objectified or formalized because they must ever be worked out anew in particular relationships and in real time. Nurses' stories illustrate this truth. Practices share social, practical, and historical bases. Excellent clinical practice requires action and reasoning in transitions with particular situations (Taylor, 1993; Benner, Tanner & Chesla, 1996; Benner, Hooper-Kyriakidis & Stannard, 1999).

Caring practices are based on meeting and responding to particular concrete others. Becoming a member-participant in nursing practice assumes a helping intent and a commitment to developing caring practices. The nurses' narratives in this book provide a moral vision for the worth and primacy of caring for healing and for rendering difficult medical cures safe and effective. One of the goals of this work is to make the caring practices that are integral to excellent nursing practice visible. Nurses' stories show how vital connections are made in the midst of busy days and multiple demands. These lessons are timeless and show how to extend and preserve our caring practices. Caring practices can be improved through better descriptive language that incorporates timing, human connections, and gains and losses in understanding across time. Organizational language and a preference for procedural descriptions of knowledge can cause caring practices to be overlooked. No one can mandate that anyone care or engage in caring practices. But nursing administrators and practicing nurses can create working environments and climates that facilitate caring practices.

Practicing nurses develop both clinical knowledge and moral agency as they learn from their patients and families. Experiential learning in high-risk situations requires courage and supportive learning environments. Nurses' stories reveal this agent-centered experiential learning. Lack of public recognition of the nature of nurses' knowledge causes nurses' clinical learning to be neglected in local practice settings.

This work was the basis of a movement to make local experiential learning public and accessible by reflecting on the clinical knowledge that is evident in narratives of experiential learning. Local practice communities develop distinct clinical knowledge and skills. Many hospitals and home nursing settings have started narrative projects to capture this local experiential knowledge. These projects systematically collect and reflect on clinical narratives of clinicians. Collecting 50 to 100 narratives of experiential learning creates a self-study of clinical knowledge that identifies strengths of practice, prevailing challenges, or silences in local practice settings. Collecting narratives and reflecting interpretively on these narratives uncovers new knowledge and skills, identifying impediments to good practice as well as areas of excellence. For example, stories may reveal remarkably strong care of the family in all settings, including the peri-operative nursing practice. Or narratives may reveal a profound silence about end-of-life care. The major goals of these narrative projects have been to make experiential clinical learning visible, collective, and cumulative. In developing a narrative account of experiential learning, the storyteller learns from telling the story. Teaching reflection allows clinicians to identify concerns that organize the story; identify notions of good embedded in the story; identify relational, communicative, and collaborative skills; and articulate newly developing clinical knowledge.

Public storytelling among practitioners makes ethical distinctions in clinical practice visible and available for evaluation. The forming of the story–what concerns shape the story and how the story ends–are revealed in the dialogue and perceptions of the storyteller. Narratives reveal context, process, and content of practical moral reasoning. Thus, stories create moral imagination even as they expose knowledge gaps and paradoxes. Practitioners' stories also demonstrate that compassion can be both wise and less costly than adversarial, commodified health care.

Aristotle noted distinctions between a practice and production or the making of things. This work allows nurses to distinguish among knowledge available from science, technology, and practice. Distinctions between technical procedural knowledge and clinical judgment or phronesis are evident in the nurses' exemplars that demonstrate clinical reasoning embedded in human relationships. In the context of current engineering and commercial models of health care, these distinctions are even more relevant. Practice is an integrated whole that requires the practitioner to develop character, knowledge, and skill in order to contribute to the development of the practice. Practice is more than a collection of techniques. Mastering specialized aspects of a practice will not necessarily qualify the practitioner to be recognized as an expert. Science and technology push the development of a practice such as nursing, but without a coherent tradition that has socially recognized standards of practice and notions of good practice, practitioners would not know how to evaluate or pursue the development of science and technologies. It is not a question of choosing *either* science *or* practical wisdom, but rather how to relate the two.

Interviewing and observing nurses for this research was transformative for me as a nurse and as an educator. This research was conducted during an acute nursing shortage and extreme budget cutbacks. Nursing educators were engaged in a competency-based education movement. This movement was designed to prespecify learning outcomes in well-defined behavioral objectives. The assumption was that both learning and nursing practice could be reduced to a collection of techniques. A technical understanding of nursing was rampant within both nursing education and practice. The phrase *technical understanding* refers to an assumption that all action can be determined through explicitly stated theories and directives. The original goal behind this research was to address the theory–practice gap. Instead, this research revealed many gaps between excellent practice and extant theoretical accounts of nursing practice. Nursing practice is far more complex than what most formal nursing theories predict. The observations and narrative interviews of practicing nurses demonstrate high levels of judgment. For example: Nurses provide life-saving early warnings about patients' clinical changes; nurses administer instantaneous therapies according to patient responses; caring practices, including healing relationships and coaching, help patients and families cope with their illnesses. It became apparent that caring practices embedded in the teaching-coaching and helping roles of nurses were essential to the success of highly technical medical interventions because they render them safe and trustworthy for patients.

Narrative accounts of experiences in nursing practice reveal major aspects of the nursing role that cannot be captured in formal descriptions of techniques and procedures, or task analyses approaches to job descriptions. Nurses often described a perceptual clarity of patient signs and symptoms based on their prior experience. This kind of certainty and clarity is distinct from the certainty of criterial reasoning, and signals the need for further assessment. Articulating the knowledge embedded in the caring and clinical practices of nurses and other healthcare workers provides one way of bringing these skilled practices in from the margins. Caring practices need to be articulated and recovered (made public so that they can be legitimized and valued) because they sustain trustworthy relationships that make health promotion, restoration, and rehabilitation possible. Caring practices cannot thrive if they continue to be undervalued. Understanding caring as a practice, rather than as pure sentiment or attitudes apart from the practice, reveals the knowledge and skill that excellent caring requires. Studying a socially organized practice allows for a collective reflection that can build knowledge and create new research agendas.

The Dreyfus Model of Skill Acquisition (Dreyfus and Dreyfus, 1986) is based on studying a practice situation by situation, and determining the level of practice evident in the situation. It elucidates strengths rather than deficits, and describes practice capacities rather than traits or talents. At each stage of experiential learning, clinicians can perform at their best. For example, one can be the best novice (typically a first-year nursing student) ever. One can be the most responsible and engaged clinical inquirer and experiential learner whatever the stage of skill acquisition. What one cannot do is be beyond experience, or be responsible for what has not yet been encountered in practice. Professionals can be held responsible for safe practice, and for knowing current science and technology. Memorizing characteristics and features of a diagnostic category from a textbook, however, is not the same as recognizing when and how these characteristics manifest themselves in particular patients, with a range of variation. This clinical discernment must be learned in practice.

Experiential learning in high-risk environments requires developing a sense of moral agency and responsibility. Experiential learning is enhanced in supportive learning communities and organizational climates. For example, a clinician who has seen only one open-heart surgery patient recover cannot be expected to make qualitative distinctions or comparisons with other recovering patients. This ability to compare whole concrete clinical cases is distinctly more nuanced and more powerful in recognizing clinical variations than can be depicted in textbooks or critical pathways. This is an obvious statement, but it is often ignored in a technical vision of practice, where it is imagined that critical pathways can make explicit the myriad trajectories and variations in patient care and recovery. Although clinicians cannot be held accountable for nuanced clinical variations that they have not seen in their practice, they can work collaboratively with their colleagues to make the best use of experientially gained clinical wisdom.

Learning to meet others in varying states of vulnerability and suffering requires openness and experiential learning over time. Keeping track of times of relative effectiveness in meeting and connecting with another can reveal and extend one's skills of engagement. Paradigm cases are highlighted in this work—clinical experiences that teach clinicians something new about practice so that their subsequent practice is changed or transformed in some way. I encourage nursing students and practicing nurses either to write or tape record their paradigm cases as a self-study of their own clinical learning over time. This is a good way to connect personal learning with professional learning. For example, learning to listen actively and respond empathetically to someone who is facing death is not easily learned. Everyone comes to such an emotionally laden situation with his or her own death anxiety and with skills of involvement learned from his or her family and from life. By recording paradigm cases in which either good rapport or breakdown in communication occurred, nurses can extend their experiential learning and self-development. Nurse educators can use first-person experience-near narratives similar to the ones presented in this book to help students to reflect on their practice, and articulate clinical knowledge. Students can write first person, experience-based narratives about clinical situations that taught them something new about practice, or that stood out in their memory for other reasons, such as mistakes made, lessons learned, or examples of the best of their practice. Students are encouraged to write with clarity, vividness, and honesty to provide the reader with enough detail to imagine the situation. Because articulating experiential learning is the goal, students may write about breakdown situations vividly, and provide reflective commentary that helps extend insights gained. Teaching courageous reflection on real experiential learning in practice requires a safe and open learning environment. The nurses' stories in this book provide a guide.

Nursing is practiced in real settings with real constraints, possibilities, and resources. Working environments may constrain one's practice beyond his or her ability to respond effectively. Nursing is a socially embedded and collectively held practice. All the narratives in this book come from a time of acute nursing shortage, when organizational directives and procedures had grown to alarming proportions. The clinical judgment required for good nursing practice was severely underestimated in each of the hospitals studied. These conditions are now replicated as nursing faces yet another acute shortage, and the health-care industry is engaged in cost-cutting strategies. The nursing narratives demonstrate how meeting particular patients or families enables nurses to respond well in less-than-ideal situations. The constraints on practice show up, and call for remedial attention. It is paradoxical that in the most distressed economic and staffing times, the need for holding open the vision of excellent nursing practice is greatest, if we wish to preserve the practice for present and future generations of patients and nurses. The nurses' stories point the way by showing what nursing as an integrated relational practice looks like.

Because excellent caring practices as well as diagnostic, monitoring, and therapeutic interventions are relational and contextual, the clinician cannot be sure whether such excellent practice could occur in other settings, relationships, or circumstances. Local specific knowledge, as well as general knowledge, is evident in every nursing story. Each has something of both the universal and the particular. Clinicians who are good clinical inquirers and who have benefited from much clinical learning will predictably perform better than nurses with less clinical knowledge in complex open-ended clinical situations. All clinicians are aided or constrained by the level of collaboration, resources, and organizational structures and processes available in the moment.

When any clinician fails to understand the ends or goals of practice, good clinical judgment is impossible, since good clinical judgment depends on seeing the good in any clinical situation and understanding how to actualize that good (Rubin, 1996). Narrow rational-technical visions of practice occlude the ends or goods in nursing. Narrow technical-rationality assumes that clinical judgment and moral agency are restricted to rationally calculating costs and benefits of a range of actions based on objective data. But clinical discernment and healing relationships cannot be reduced to rational calculations about subjective symptoms and objective signs. Good clinical judgment requires that clinicians envision relevant worthy ends in any patient encounter. This requires meeting the patient as a person first, and secondly as a person with particular strengths and vulnerabilities. The nurses' clinical narratives in this book continue to provide a powerful moral vision of such excellent nursing practice.

| Contents

Contents

Contents

| Preface

This book is based on a dialogue with nurses and nursing, descriptive research that identified five levels of competency in clinical nursing practice. These levels — novice, advanced beginner, competent, proficient, and expert — are described in the words of nurses who were interviewed and observed either individually or in small groups. Only patient care situations where the nurse made a positive difference in the patient's outcome are included. These situations offer vivid examples of excellence in actual nursing practice. They are not abstract ideals, however; they emerge from the imperfections and contingencies with which nurses work daily.

A Note to the Skeptics

Some who read the exemplars will be skeptical that such nursing is possible. Their skepticism is warranted, because these examples are drawn from outstanding clinical situations where the nurse learned something about her practice or made a significant contribution to a patient's welfare. But if the reader's skepticism stems from a generalized disillusionment with nursing in hospitals and from the belief that nurses are rendered impotent to give compassionate, lifesaving care in hospitals — then this book offers a resounding rebuttal to the skeptic and a ray of hope to the disillusioned.

The Perceptual Origins of Excellence

This book questions some of nursing's most dearly held beliefs and assumptions. The book asserts that perceptual awareness is central to good nursing judgment and that this begins with vague hunches and global assessments that initially bypass critical analysis; conceptual clarity follows more often than it precedes. Experienced nurses often describe their perceptual abilities using phrases such as "gut feeling," a "sense of uneasiness," or a "feeling that things are not quite right." This kind of talk makes educators and clinicians uncomfortable, because the assessment must move from these perceptual beginnings to conclusive evidence. Expert nurses know that in all cases definitive evaluation of a patient's condition requires more than vague hunches, but through experience they have learned to allow their perceptions to lead to confirming evidence.

In the quest for a scientific rationale, the importance of perceptual skills can be overlooked by any clinician — nurse, physician, or counselor. If nurses were disembodied computers or mechanical monitoring devices, they would have to wait for clear, explicit signals before identifying one singular feature of a problem. Fortunately, however, expert human decision makers can get a gestalt of the situation and proceed to follow up on vague, subtle changes in the patient's condition with a confirmatory search aided by the whole health care team. Experts dare not stop with vague hunches, but neither do they dare to ignore those hunches that could lead to early identification of problems and the search for confirming evidence.

| The Importance of Discretionary Judgment

Considering the early history of nursing education in this country, I am concerned that the model of skill acquisition described here could be misinterpreted as advocating informal trial-and-error learning. Therefore, it is important to point out that the Dreyfus Model of Skill Acquisition was originally developed in research designed to study pilots' performance in emergency situations. In that context, no one worried that people might misinterpret the model and suggest that the pilot should just go out and "get the feel of the plane" through trial and error; under those circumstances the beginning pilot would not even survive basic training. The same holds true for nursing. Providing nursing care involves risks for both nurse and patient, and skilled nursing requires well-planned educational programs. Experience-based skill acquisition is safer and quicker when it rests upon a sound educational base.

This book's purpose is to present the limits of formal rules and call attention to the discretionary judgment used in actual clinical situations. This does not place the expert in a special, privileged position outside the principles of physiology, nursing, and medicine. The book does not advocate a chaotic or anarchical position that would claim there are no rules — that would confer a license, for instance, to ignore the rules of asepsis simply because sterile technique must be sometimes ignored in life-and-death emergencies. Attending to the particular contingencies of a situation does not warrant the conclusion that the general principles governing that situation can be generally ignored. My position is not a careless recommendation for the abandonment of rules. Instead, I am claiming that a more skilled, advanced understanding of the situation allows orderly behavior without rigid rule following.

Once the situation is described, the actions taken can be understood as orderly, reasonable behavior that responds to the demands of a given situation rather than rigid principles and rules. More descriptive rules could be generated to allow for multiple exceptions, but the expert would still function flexibly in other new situations requiring new exceptions. The book addresses the risky, situation-specific decisions that are usually covered up but that nurses face daily in their practice. Menzies (1960) referred to hiding behind rules and policies as a defense against anxiety, a coping strategy. But as a coping strategy it is unrealistic and creates the additional burden of lack of recognition and legitimization of actual nursing performance.

| Reflecting the Realities of Practice

Readers would probably prefer that I had chosen only exemplars reflecting ideal collaborative behaviors and ideal relationships with physicians. In fact, nursing administrators and physicians have warned me that they do not like the exemplars showing the doctor–nurse relationship in a bad light. I, too, wish that in conducting this study I had found only enlightened, collaborative relationships between nurses and physicians, but that would have been fiction and not descriptive research — an ideal model instead of an empirically tested one. If there is a bias, it is probably in the other direction: that troubled nurse–physician exchanges are *under-represented*, given the amount of interview time nurses spent describing troubled interactions.

In the real world, nurses and physicians alike have good and bad days; some are frankly incompetent. When immediate physician attention to a crisis is not available, the nurse fills the gap far more often than is formally acknowledged. We can claim that this is not nursing, but we do so only by ignoring what nurses actually do. Therefore, skilled performance was considered excellent because, even lacking the best of circumstances (e.g., collaborative relationships or formally acknowledged nursing functions), the nurse procured or did what was needed for the patient. By attending to the ideal and presenting only what we hope to become, we would miss much of what is significant about our actual practice. Not knowing who and what we are about *now* will seriously impede what we want to become.

A Kaleidoscope of Intimacy and Distance

The reader would be correct to question the representativeness of this work. The goal was not to describe a typical day or hour but rather the highlights, the growing edges of clinical knowledge. The participants were asked to present clinical situations that stood out in their minds. Nurses make many contacts with patients daily; most of the time they are unaware of the impact their interventions have on the patient's recovery. Many of these contacts and interventions are routine and not even remembered by the nurses. In other words, the nurse–patient relationship is not a uniform professionalized blueprint but rather a kaleidoscope of intimacy and distance in some of the most dramatic, poignant, and mundane moments of life. The mundane moments were not captured because this research strategy asked specifically for outstanding clinical situations. So this bias remains, even though we asked for descriptions of both typical and unusual days. Since we sought to describe skilled performance, deficits were not the point of inquiry, so there are no negative examples of deficits identified (see Fenton, pp. 262–74 for an example of identification of deficits).

Not an End but a Beginning

I am concerned about hasty system builders who will want to deify the 31 competencies described or who might want to complete the list, as though there were a finite list of competencies that can be captured for all time. Ending with 31 is indeed a bit whimsical, but the intent of this work is to encourage nurses to collect their *own* exemplars and to pursue the lines of inquiry and research questions raised by their *own* clinical knowledge. This work presents new ways to view nursing practice so that we do not continue to limit the description of such practice to a simplified, linear, problem-solving process. Such uniformity and constriction limit our understanding of the complexity and significance of our practice. As one nurse said with a note of realization, in a group discussion: "You know, I acted very quickly and saved a baby's life today. That's not insignificant!" It seemed that she had failed to take account of the import of her actions in her earlier analytical reporting.

I am grateful to colleagues who have enriched this work by providing descriptions — an early map, so to speak — of the practical applications of this work (see Epilogue).

This work came out of a federally funded training grant to develop methods of evaluation for seven participating schools of nursing and five hospitals in the San Francisco Bay Area. The title of the project grant was Achieving Methods of Intra-professional Consensus, Assessment, and Evaluation, hereafter referred to as the AMICAE Project. Support for this project was provided by a grant from the Department of Health and Human Services, Public Health Service, Division of Nursing, Grant No. 7 D10 NU 29104-01.

Patricia Benner

| Acknowledgments

This book is based on a community effort, so any attempt to acknowledge all the contributions will necessarily fall short. I am indebted to all those who gave us access and made it easier to contact over 1,200 nurses through questionnaires and interviews. The study would not have been possible without the ten-year tradition of cooperation between nursing service and nursing education, fostered by the San Francisco Committee on Nursing and Nursing Education under the guidance of Dr. Helen Nahm. I am grateful to all directors of nursing in the participating hospitals and to the deans of the participating schools of nursing for making this research possible.

The staff on the AMICAE Project have also significantly contributed to this research. Ruth Colavecchio, Deborah Gordon, and Judith Wrubel all assisted with the interviews and the interview analysis. Deborah Gordon conducted extensive observation and interviewing on two acute general surgical units. Ruth Colavecchio worked with one of the participating hospitals in developing a ladder of clinical promotion, based upon the Dreyfus Model of Skill Acquisition applied to nursing. Kathy Field's dedication and interest in the effort to describe nursing competencies in a new way made the contact transcription and retrieval of interviews and field notes possible. She also typed the manuscript and provided editorial assistance. Denise Henjum typed transcripts of many hours of interviews.

A special note of thanks is due to Professors Hubert L. and Stuart E. Dreyfus who provided expert consultation on applying their model to clinical nursing practice.

I also wish to express appreciation to the many nurses who participated in this study. I hope that this book will serve as tribute to both the beginning and experienced nurses who willingly and diligently described and allowed us to observe their practice. It is primarily their story that is told in the following pages. Their descriptions of patient care situations where they made a difference well represent nursing expertise and commitment. They present the uniqueness of nursing as a discipline and an art, as no other descriptive strategy could. The themes of patient advocacy, expertise, and involvement that create vigilance and comprise caring are repeated throughout these nurses' stories.

I am grateful to Edith (Pat) Lewis for her immeasurable help in the creation of this book. Her intimate knowledge of the field of nursing enabled her to grasp the larger significance of the work and steer it in the right direction through perceptive editing.

I am indebted to the people of Addison-Wesley, particularly Nancy Evans, Senior Editor, and Jan deProsse, Production Coordinator, who gave expert guidance in turning a monograph into a book. Their quick responses, dedication to excellence, and interest in the content contributed greatly to this work.

Finally, I would like to thank the following persons for reviewing the manuscript before publication and contributing their helpful suggestions: Kathleen Fischer, University of Michigan Hospitals; Marian Langer and Mary Hutchings, St. John's Hospital, St. Louis; Sydney Krampitz, University of Kansas; Shirley Martin, University of Missouri; Rosalyn Jazwiec and Teresa Tapella, Northwestern Memorial Hospital.

P.B.

1 | Uncovering the Knowledge Embedded in Clinical Nursing Practice*

Nursing practice has been studied primarily from a sociological perspective. Thus, we have learned much about role relationships, socialization, and acculturation in nursing practice. But, we have learned less about the knowledge embedded in actual nursing practice — i.e., that knowledge that accrues over time in the practice of an applied discipline. Such knowledge has gone uncharted and unstudied because the differences between practical and theoretical knowledge have been misunderstood (Carper, 1978; Collins & Fielder, 1981). What's missing are systematic observations of what nurse clinicians learn from their clinical practice.

Nurses have not been careful record keepers of their own clinical learning. Although many single case studies have been published, few clinical comparisons of multiple case studies or clinical observations across

*This chapter is adapted, with permission, from an article by the author ("Uncovering the Knowledge Embedded in Clinical Practice") that was published in *Image: The Journal of Nursing Scholarship,* Vol. XV, No. 2, Spring 1983.

patient populations exist. This failure to chart our practices and clinical observations has deprived nursing theory of the uniqueness and richness of the knowledge embedded in expert clinical practice. Well-charted practices and observations are essential for theory development.

This book will examine the differences between practical and theoretical knowledge; provide examples of competencies identified from the study of nursing practice; describe aspects of practical knowledge; and outline strategies for preserving and extending that knowledge. First, however, let us take an overall look at the nature of that knowledge and how it is acquired.

Differences Between Practical and Theoretical Knowledge

Theory is a powerful tool for explaining and predicting. It shapes questions and allows the systematic examination of a series of events. Theorists try to identify the necessary and sufficient conditions for the occurrence of real situations. By establishing interactional causal relationships between events, scientists come to "know that." Philosophers of science such as Kuhn (1970) and Polanyi (1958), however, observe that "knowing *that*" and "knowing *how*" are two different kinds of knowledge. They point out that we have many skills (know how) that are acquired without "knowing *that*" and, further, that we cannot always theoretically account for our know-how for many common activities such as riding a bicycle or swimming. To state it differently, some practical knowledge may elude scientific formulations of "knowing that." And "know-how" that may challenge or extend current theory can be developed ahead of such scientific formulations. Therefore, knowledge development in an applied discipline consists of extending practical knowledge (know-how) through theory-based scientific investigations and through the charting of the existent "know-how" developed through clinical experience in the practice of that discipline.

Knowledge Embedded in Expertise

Expertise develops when the clinician tests and refines propositions, hypotheses, and principle-based expectations in actual practice situations. Experience, as it is used here (Heidegger, 1962; Gadamer, 1970), results when preconceived notions and expectations are challenged, refined, or disconfirmed by the actual situation. Experience is therefore a requisite for expertise. For example, the problem solving of a proficient or expert nurse differs from that of the beginner or competent nurse, as described in Chapter 2. This difference can be attributed to the know-how that is acquired through experience. The expert nurse perceives the situation as a whole, uses past concrete situations as paradigms, and moves to the accurate region of the problem without wasteful consideration of a large number of irrelevant options (Dreyfus, H., 1979; Dreyfus, S., 1981). In contrast, the competent or proficient nurse in a novel situation must rely on conscious, deliberate, analytic problem solving of an elemental nature.

Expertise in complex human decision making, such as nursing requires, makes the interpretation of clinical situations possible, and the knowledge embedded in this clinical expertise is central to the advancement of nursing practice and the development of nursing science. Not all of the knowledge embedded in expertise can be captured in theoretical propositions, or with analytic strategies that depend on identifying all the elements that go into the decision (Benner & Benner, 1979). However, the intentions, expectations, meanings, and outcomes of expert practice can be described, and aspects of clinical know-how can be captured by interpretive descriptions of actual practice.

Extending Practical Knowledge

Clinical knowledge is gained over time, and clinicians themselves are often unaware of their gains. Strategies are needed to make clinical know-how public so it can be extended and refined. Six areas of practical knowledge were identified: (1) graded qualitative distinctions; (2) common meanings; (3) assumptions, expectations, and sets; (4) paradigm cases and personal knowledge; (5) maxims; and (6) unplanned practices. Each area can be studied using ethnographic and interpretive strategies intitally to identify and extend practical knowledge.

Expert nurses, for instance, learn to recognize subtle physiological changes. They can recognize signs of impending shock before documentable changes in vital signs are apparent and can discriminate the need for imminent resuscitation efforts prior to vascular collapse or dramatic vital sign change. Many examples of early recognition and early warnings by expert nurses are documented in this book—e.g., pulmonary embolus, or early stages of septic shock. These finely tuned abilities come from many hours of direct patient observation and care.

Often the perceptual grasp of a situation is context dependent; that is, the subtle changes take on significance only in light of the patient's past history and current situation. Polanyi (1958) calls this perceptual, recognitional ability of the expert clinician, "connoisseurship." Descriptive and interpretive recording of this connoisseurship uncovers clinical knowledge. Nurses need to collect examples of their recognitional abilities and describe the context, meanings, characteristics, and outcomes of their connoisseurship. This will enable them to refine their skills and to demonstrate or illustrate the qualitative distinctions they have come to recognize. Much of this takes place naturally as nurses compare their judgments of qualitative distinctions such as tonicity in a premature infant or the "feel" of a contracted uterus in contrast to one that is firm because of clots.

Graded qualitative distinctions can be elaborated and refined only as nurses compare their judgments in actual patient care situations. For example, intensive care nursery nurses compare their assessments of muscle tone so that they can come to consistent appraisals of tonicity. Nurses evaluating wound healing compare their descriptive language as patient examples present themselves. Often, special descriptive terms will develop to describe these qualitative distinctions. However, unless steps are taken to systematically compare the meaning of these terms in actual situations, communication will break down.

This aspect of clinical knowledge (connoisseurship) is often overlooked in the quest to learn the latest technological procedures. An inordinate amount of attention is given to learning the latest technology and procedures rather than to in-depth skill acquisition in clinical judgment.

Common Meanings

As illustrated in the competencies presented in Chapters 4 and 5, nurses working with common issues in health and illness, birth and death, develop common meanings about helping, recovering, and coping resources in these human situations. For example, one common meaning uncovered in this study is that nurses typically try to develop a sense of "possibility" for their patients even in the most deprived circumstances and even when this sense of possibility may mean only a pain-free afternoon or even acceptance of pain or death.

Nurses learn from families and patients a range of responses, meanings, and coping options in the most extreme situations. These common meanings evolve over time and are shared among nurses. They form a tradition. Understanding these meanings *without* rendering them meaningless through decontextualized analysis can provide a seedbed for systematic study and the further development of practice and theory. Common meanings become apparent when narrative accounts of diverse clinical situations are given with the intentions, context, and meanings intact.

Assumptions, Expectations, and Sets

Accounts of practical situations presented in narrative form with the context intact are laden with assumptions, expectations, and "sets" that may not be a part of formally recognized knowledge. When a narrative account is examined for the assumptions and expectations underlying the assessment or interventions, new questions can be generated for further refinement, development, and testing. For example, from having observed the clinical course of many similar and dissimilar patients, nurses may learn to expect a certain course of events without ever formally stating those expectations. These expectations may show up only in clinical practice and not in known abstractions or generalizations.

Nurses also develop global sets about patients. Gestalt psychologists define "set" as a predisposition to act in certain ways in particular situations. Sets are accrued over time and may be even more elusive than the specific expectations or assumptions that are often apparent to the outside observer. Sets constitute the orientation toward the situation and thus alter how the situation is perceived and described. Sets can sometimes be uncovered, though they can never be completely explicit because the very act of making them explicit will change their function.

One strategy for making sets more visible is borrowed from cross-cultural studies where different "sets" for the same situation become apparent when communication breaks down or actions do not make sense to people with divergent cultural backgrounds. Deliberate cross-cultural experiments can be created through nurses' comparing critical incidents from their practice and the ways in which they approach a clinical situation.

Divergent approaches and breakdowns in communication about the same clinical situation may point to different sets. For example, different sets were apparent in two nurses' descriptions of identifying and managing a patient crisis until physician assistance was available. One nurse had worked in a setting where nurse-physician trust and communication were high, whereas the other nurse worked in a setting where distrust was the norm and physicians even refused to sign verbal orders. Consequently, the nurse working in the latter setting did not approach a medically urgent patient situation with the same set or sense of possibility as the nurse working in the highly collaborative setting. Discovering assumptions, expectations, and sets can uncover an unexamined area of practical knowledge that can then be systematically studied and extended or refuted.

Paradigm Cases and Personal Knowledge

Heidegger (1962) and Gadamer (1975) define experience as the turning around of preconceptions that are not confirmed by the actual situation. The precondition for perceiving a situation is a foreknowledge or set, and in clinical practice this foreknowledge is often well formed by theory, principles, and prior experience. Only when the event refines, elaborates, or disconfirms this foreknowledge does the event deserve the term "experience." As a nurse gains "experience," clinical knowledge that is a hybrid between naive practical knowledge and unrefined theoretical knowledge develops. A particular experience may be powerful enough to stand out as a paradigm case (Benner & Wrubel, 1982). Many of the exemplars presented in later chapters were paradigm cases for the nurses who presented them.

Proficient and expert nurses develop clusters of paradigm cases around different patient care issues (see Chapter 2, pp. 27–36), so that they approach a patient care situation using past concrete situations much as a researcher uses a paradigm. Past situations stand out because they changed the nurse's perception. Past concrete experience therefore guides the expert's perceptions and actions and allows for a rapid perceptual grasp of the situation. This kind of advanced clinical knowledge is more comprehensive than any theoretical sketch can be, since the proficient clinician compares past whole situations with current whole situations.

Some paradigm cases are sufficiently simple and dramatic that they can be transmitted as case studies and taken up as paradigms by the learner (Benner & Wrubel, 1982). Expert clinical teachers present paradigm cases that transmit more than can be conveyed through abstract principles or guidelines. But in order for students to learn from another person's paradigm case, they must actively rehearse or imagine the situation. Simulations can be even more effective because they require action and decisions from the learner. In addition, simulations provide the learner with opportunities to gain paradigm cases in a guided way.

However, many paradigm cases are too complex to be transmitted through case examples or simulations, because it is the particular interaction with the individual learner's prior knowledge that creates the "experience" — that is, the particular refinement or turning around of preconceptions and prior understanding. Polanyi (1958) calls this a transaction with personal knowledge. Each person brings his own particular history, intellectual commitments, and readiness to learn to a particular clinical situation. The transactions created by this personal knowledge and the clinical situation then determine the actions and decisions that are made. This is why a clinical discipline needs expert clinicians to model this dynamic transaction between personal knowledge and the clinical situation.

Experienced nurses can readily bring to mind clinical situations that altered their approach to patient care. Through a systematic record and study of these para-

9

digm cases, it is possible to extend the knowledge that is embedded there.

Maxims

Experts pass on cryptic instructions that make sense only if the person already has a deep understanding of the situation. Polanyi (1958) calls these instructions "maxims" (Dreyfus, 1982; Benner, 1982; Benner & Wrubel, 1982). For example, intensive care nurses point cryptically to subtle changes in premature infants' respiratory status that will make sense only to one who has had a range of experience in observing respiratory status in premature infants. Polanyi (1958) uses the example of maxims in sports. The experienced golfer or tennis player is told to "keep your eye on the ball," whereas it would make no sense to give the beginner the same message.

Expert nurse clinicians can learn much from the maxims they are able to pass on to one another. However, the outside observer and less expert nurse can also gain clues about areas of clinical knowledge — particularly perceptual knowledge that is cloaked in maxims. Collecting maxims can be a beginning point for identifying an area of clinical judgment.

Unplanned Practices

The nursing role in hospitals and extended care facilities has expanded largely through unplanned practices and interventions delegated by the physician and other health care workers. This unplanned delegation might be termed delegation by default. For example, a new

treatment or diagnostic regimen is introduced and because of the element of risk involved, the treatment or
regimen must be administered and monitored by physicians. But frequently the nurse is given the responsibility for doing this because it is the nurse who is present
at the patient's bedside.

These handed-down practices have multiple ramifi-
cations for nursing practice. For example, nurses have
become experts in titrating and weaning patients from
vasopressors and antiarrhythmic drugs, but this knowledge has not been systematically described or studied.
Perceptions and clinical judgments are altered as a result of acquiring a new skill, yet these changes will
continue to go undocumented and unrecognized unless
nurses study these changes and the resultant "know-
how" that develops in their own practice.

Summary and Conclusions

A wealth of untapped knowledge is embedded in the
practices and the "know-how" of expert nurse clinicians, but this knowledge will not expand or fully develop unless nurses systematically record what they
learn from their own experience. Clinical expertise has
not been adequately described or compensated in nursing, and the lag in description contributes to the lag in
recognition and reward. Furthermore, adequate description of practical knowledge is essential to the development and extension of nursing theory. Nursing
science has much to gain from nurses who compare
their graded qualitative judgments and who describe
and document their observations, sets, paradigm cases,

maxims, and their changing practices. There is much to learn and appreciate as practicing nurses uncover common meanings acquired as a result of helping, coaching, and intervening in the significantly human events that comprise the art and science of nursing.

2 | The Dreyfus Model of Skill Acquisition Applied to Nursing

Stuart Dreyfus, a mathematician and system analyst, and Hubert Dreyfus, a philosopher, have developed a model of skill acquisition based upon the study of chess players and airline pilots. The Dreyfus model (Dreyfus & Dreyfus, 1980; Dreyfus, 1981) posits that in the acquisition and development of a skill, a student passes through five levels of proficiency: novice, advanced beginner, competent, proficient, and expert. These different levels reflect changes in three general aspects of skilled performance. One is a movement from reliance on abstract principles to the use of past concrete experience as paradigms. The second is a change in the learner's perception of the demand situation, in which the situation is seen less and less as a compilation of equally relevant bits, and more and more as a complete whole in which only certain parts are relevant. The third is a passage from *detached* observer to *involved* performer. The performer no longer stands outside the situation but is now engaged *in* the situation. Reported here are the results of a systematic study of the applicability of this model to nursing. Skill

13

and skilled practices are terms that will be used synonymously; both include skilled nursing interventions and clinical judgment skills. In no case are they used to mean psychomotor skills or other enabling skills demonstrable in a skills laboratory outside the normal context of practice. Thus, skills and skilled practices refer to the applied skill of nursing in actual clinical situations.

Methods

In order to ascertain and understand the differences in clinical performance and situation appraisal of beginning and expert nurses, paired interviews were conducted with beginning nurses and nurses recognized for their expertise. These nurses (21 pairs) were selected from three hospitals where preceptors are used to orient newly graduated nurses. Each member of the pair—preceptors and newly graduated nurses—was interviewed separately about patient care situations they had had in common and that stood out for them. Both were asked for the clinical knowledge that they found to be particularly difficult to teach or to learn. The research was aimed at discovering if there were distinguishable, characteristic differences in the novice's and expert's descriptions of the same clinical incident. If so, how could these differences, if identifiable from the nurses' descriptions of the incidents, be accounted for or understood?

In addition to the preceptor–preceptee paired descriptions of the same clinical incidents, interviews and/or participant observations were conducted with 51 additional experienced nurse clinicians, 11 newly graduated nurses, and 5 senior nursing students to further delineate and describe characteristics of nurse performance at different stages of skill acquisition. The interviews (small group and individual) and the participant observations were conducted in six hospitals: two private community hospitals, two community teaching hospitals, one university medical center, and one inner-city general hospital.

The 51 experienced nurses were selected by staff development directors who conferred with head nurses and peers. They were instructed to select nurses with at least five years of clinical experience currently engaged in direct patient care, and who were recognized as being highly skilled clinicians. Seven of these nurses had master's degrees, the majority had a baccalaureate; however, educational background was not a formal criterion for selection.

No attempt was made to classify the nurses themselves according to the proficiency levels; rather, each clinical situation was judged independently as reflecting a particular level of practice. This is in keeping with the nature of the Dreyfus model, which offers no context-free criteria to identify persons as possessing talents or traits indicative of expertise. This was not a search for the omnicompetent individual who could perform equally well, regardless of circumstances or educational preparation.

A series of four two-hour, small group interviews were held with four to eight experienced nurses from different patient care units within the same hospital. The schedules varied from daily interviews to biweekly interviews. Individual interviews were conducted with all 51 experienced nurses, and participant observations were made on 26 of them. In all cases, participation was minimal — limited to occasionally assisting the nurses in transporting patients and other minor tasks to make observation less intrusive and awkward. Prior to the interview sessions the participants were given a written outline of the kinds of clinical descriptions we were interested in (see Appendix A for the "critical incident" guide). With experience we learned that the research term, "critical incident," was an unfortunate label because it triggered thoughts of critical patients and crisis events. We had to explain that we were interested in significant noncrisis events as well.

The interviews were conducted by the author, a nurse researcher-administrator, a graduate student in anthropology, and a research psychologist. The interviews were tape recorded, and verbatim transcripts were made for textual analysis. In all but one of the small group interview series, at least two of the researchers were present to facilitate group process.

Interpretation of Data

The interviews and participant/observer records were read independently by the research team members, and interpretations of the data were compared and consensually validated. Each interpretation was accepted only if there was agreement in labeling and interpreting the major competency demonstrated and only if it was effective in describing skilled practice.

The interpretive strategy used was based on Heideggerian phenomenology (Heidegger, 1962; Palmer, 1969; Benner, in press), which fits the description of constant comparative method by Strauss and Glaser (Glaser, 1978; Glaser & Strauss, 1967; Wilson, 1977). However, unlike the Strauss and Glaser approach, the intent was not to come up with theoretical terms but rather to identify meanings and content.

The following interview excerpts illustrate paired descriptions of the same incident by a beginning nurse and an experienced one. The latter described an emergency clinical situation in the ICU:

I had worked late and was just about ready to go home, when a nurse preceptor said to me, "Jolene, come here." Her voice had urgency in it, but not Code Blue. I walked in and I looked at the patient and his heart rate was about 120, and he was on the respirator and breathing. And I asked her: "What's wrong?" There was a new graduate taking care of him. And he just pointed down to the patient who was lying in a pool of blood. There was a big stream of blood drooling out of his mouth. This man's diagnosis was mandibular cancer which had been resected, and about a week previous to that he had had a carotid bleed from the external carotid which had been ligated secondary to radiation erosion. That wound had become septic and he had developed respiratory failure and he was in ICU for that. So I looked at the dressing and it was dry, the blood was coming out of his mouth. The man had a tracheostomy because of the type of surgery that had been done. He also had an N.G. tube in for feedings, and I got to thinking that it might be the innominate or the carotid artery that had eroded. So we took him off the ventilator to see if anything was going to pump out of the trach. There was a little blood, but it looked mostly like it had come down from the pharynx into the lungs. So we began hand ventilating him, trying to figure out what the devil was inside his mouth that was pumping out this tremendous amount of blood. . . .

Upon questioning, the expert clinician pointed out that hand ventilation was important because it ensured that 100 percent oxygen was delivered and made it possible to feel the degree of resistance in the lungs.

Note that for this expert the problem grasp began in the hall on the way to the room. She had already picked up the fact that while the nurse's voice had urgency in it, it was not of a Code Blue urgency nature. This kind of orientation to the problem can come only with prior experience. After concluding that the problem was the carotid and not the innominate artery, applying pressure to the carotid area, and continuing with hand ventilation, the expert nurse noted:

By this time the problem is blood, we need blood, and so I said, "OK, someone call the blood bank and get some blood." And the nurse said, "We just called and there's none down there." No one had caught that the patient was sitting up there with no blood in the blood bank. So we took off a blood from the arterial line and sent it down for a type and cross match. Meanwhile, I started Plasmanate and lactated Ringers, because the mean pressure was dropping down to about 30 and the blood was just pumping out of his mouth.

Interviewer: Were there any physicians on the scene at this point?

Expert Nurse: They had been called but had not arrived yet. But about this time the ICU resident came in and looked bewildered like "what are we going to do?" He asked if we had an ancillary line in. I said, "Yes, we have a central venous pressure line in, but I don't think that's going to be enough." He said, "I'll do a cutdown." I said, "I don't think you have to; I think I can get one in." So I took a 14-gauge and put it into the intracubital space. There are two plasmas going in. He said, "What shall I do?" And I said, "You need to go down to the blood bank and get some type-specific blood for this patient, because a nurse can't get that. You are the only person who can get type-specific blood." I said, "Bring two units; they will only give you two at a time, no matter how bad. But bring two and get back here as soon as you can." So he took off.

The patient's fluid resuscitation was successful and the bleeding was controlled enough to get the patient to surgery in time to repair the artery.

With the expert's account the listener is placed deep into the situation; one forgets who is telling the story, which is only as detailed as it needs to be for other nurses to grasp what's going on. There are no extraneous details except when the listeners needed clarification on a technical issue. The expert is at home with the language; she talks fluently about the mean blood pressure. She used her hand to illustrate how the ventilatory bag feels when she is checking the lung resistance. She knows in her hands how different resistances feel, so she uses gestures to convey these differences. These points are best illustrated by contrasting them with an advanced beginner's description of the same situation.

This man is a very pleasant fellow, very bright, very alert and awake, and was unfortunately requiring tracheal suctioning approximately every hour to two hours for moderate amounts of tracheal secretions which were relatively tenacious in character, relatively white tannish in color. He unfortunately did not tolerate the suctioning extremely well. It was relatively uncomfortable for him, caused a moderate amount of cough and gag reflex, which in turn caused a transient increase in blood pressure. Following suctioning on one occasion, as I was replacing his tracheal mist mask, he began coughing up very copious amounts of bright red blood per mouth. I mildly panicked, called for help from the nurse next door, placed him in a moderate Trendelenberg position, opened his I.V. to a rapid rate, and continued to experience mild panic. Perhaps more like moderate panic.

Although the advanced beginner in this situation performed extremely well for his level of proficiency, his description of the situation is presented through the screen of his anxiety. The situation does not stand out as clearly as in the expert's description. There is a "subtext" of questioning whether he, the nurse, may have actually caused the carotid rupture by too traumatic suctioning. He has no way of judging what is too traumatic, so he gives a history of the suctioning with the implicit question: Could this have led to the rupture of the carotid?

With this nurse's account one can smell the textbook; he is not yet at home with the language, and the words sound like foreign objects. He uses extraneous words and gives extraneous information. His grasp of the unfolding situation is not as complete and forward looking as is the expert's. The expert seems to be one step ahead in mobilizing the resources available and in meeting the next contingency.

Through analysis of this and all the other situations that were described, and following the Dreyfus model, it became possible to describe the performance characteristics at each level of development and to identify, in general terms, the teaching/learning needs at each level.

Stage 1: Novice

Beginners have had no experience of the situations in which they are expected to perform. To give them entry to these situations and allow them to gain the experience so necessary for skill development, they are taught about the situations in terms of objective attributes such as weight, intake and output, temperature, blood pressure, pulse, and other such objectifiable, measurable parameters of a patient's condition — features of the task world that can be recognized without situational experience. Novices are also taught context-free rules to guide action in respect to different attributes. For instance:

> To determine fluid balance, check the patient's morning weights and daily intake and output for the past three days. Weight gain and an intake that is consistently higher than output by greater than 500 cc. could indicate water retention, in which case fluid restriction should be started until the cause of the imbalance can be determined.

The rule-governed behavior typical of the novice is extremely limited and inflexible. The heart of the difficulty lies in the fact that since novices have no experience of the situation they face, they must be given rules to guide their performance. But following rules legislates *against* successful performance because the rules cannot tell them the most relevant tasks to perform in an actual situation.

Nursing students enter a new clinical area as novices; they have little understanding of the contextual meaning of the recently learned textbook terms. But students are not the only novices; any nurse entering a clinical setting where she or he has no experience with the patient population may be limited to the novice level of performance if the goals and tools of patient care are unfamiliar.

This point illustrates the situational, experience-based premises of the Dreyfus model, which distinguishes between the level of skilled performance that can be achieved through principles and theory learned in a classroom and the context-dependent judgments and skill that can be acquired only in real situations (Dreyfus, 1982). For example, a clinical specialist

21

with graduate work and in-depth experience in adult critical care would be at the novice stage of skilled performance were she or he to transfer to a neonatal intensive care unit. As previously emphasized, the Dreyfus model of skill acquisition is a situational model rather than a trait or talent model.

Stage 2: Advanced Beginner

Advanced beginners are ones who can demonstrate marginally acceptable performance, ones who have coped with enough real situations to note (or to have pointed out to them by a mentor) the recurring meaningful situational components that are termed "aspects of the situation" in the Dreyfus model.

Aspects, in contrast to the measurable, context-free attributes or the procedural lists of things to do that are learned and used by the beginner, require prior experience in actual situations for recognition. Aspects include overall, global characteristics that can be identified only through prior experience. For example, assessing the patient's readiness to learn depends on experience with previous patients with similar teaching-learning needs. An expert clinician describes her assessment of a patient's readiness to learn about his ileostomy this way:

Earlier I thought he was feeling helpless about the operation he had just had. He looked as though he felt crummy—physically, sort of stressed-looking, nervous-looking. Furthermore, he was treating the wound physically very gingerly. He didn't need to be that gentle with it. But on this morning, it was different; he began to ask questions about his care.

22

Implications for Teaching and Learning

The instructor can provide guidelines for recognizing such aspects as a patient's readiness to learn. For example, "Notice whether or not the patient asks questions about the surgery or the dressing change." "Observe whether or not the patient looks at or handles the wound." But these guidelines depend on the practitioner's knowing what these aspects sound and look like in actual patient care situations. Thus, while aspects may be made explicit, they cannot be made completely objective. The nurse can gain cues from the way that the patient asks about the surgery or the dressing change, but no one cue is definitive in all situations. Experience is needed before the nurse can apply the guidelines to individual patients.

The advanced beginner or that person's instructor can now formulate principles that dictate actions in terms of both attributes and aspects. These principles, which presuppose experience-based, meaningful elements, are called guidelines. The guidelines integrate as many attributes and aspects as possible, but they tend to ignore their differential importance; i.e., they treat all attributes and aspects as equally important. This is illustrated in the following comments from an expert nurse about advanced beginners in an intensive care nursery:

I give instructions to the new graduate, very detailed and explicit instructions: When you come in and first see the baby, you take the baby's vital signs and make the physical examination, and you check the I.V. sites, and the ventilator and make sure that it works, and you check the monitors and alarms. When I would say this to them, they would do exactly what I told them to do, no matter what else was going on . . . they couldn't choose one to leave out. They couldn't choose which was the most important . . . They couldn't do for one baby the things that were most important and then go to the other baby and do the things that were most important, and leave out the things that weren't as important until later on.

Novices and advanced beginners can take in little of the situation: it is too new, too strange, and besides, they have to concentrate on remembering the rules they have been taught. The expert clinician just quoted goes on to note:

If I said, you have to do these eight things . . . they did those things, and they didn't care if their other kid was screaming its head off. When they did realize, they would be like a mule between two piles of hay.

Much time is spent by preceptors and new nurses on aspect recognition. In making physical assessments, for example, aspect recognition is an appropriate learning goal. The nurse will practice discriminating between normal, hyperactive, and missing bowel sounds on a postsurgical patient. But in practice areas where the clinician has already attained competency, aspect recognition will probably be redundant, and it will be possible to focus on the more advanced clinical skill of judging the relative importance of different aspects of the situation.

The major implication here for both preservice and staff education is that advanced beginners need support in the clinical setting. They need help, for instance, in setting priorities, since they operate on general guidelines and are only beginning to perceive recurrent meaningful patterns in their clinical practice. Their nursing care of patients needs to be backed up by nurses who have reached at least the competent level of skill and performance, to ensure that important patient needs do not go unattended because the advanced beginner cannot yet sort out what is most important. This need is illustrated by a preceptor's description of a newly graduated nurse's performance:

> In the beginning it was one thing, almost to the exclusion of everything else with the patient. For example, an EKG was done, and I found that the patient was having premature ventricular contractions, and that the doctor should be notified. *Well,* everything came to a screeching halt while he (the nurse) stopped and looked at the EKG, and he wanted me to explain an EKG and how you read them. And at this point there were still at least three other urgent patient needs to be met. It was valid for him to learn, but there was simply no time to stop everything and focus on the EKG strip.

In orienting the neophyte nurse, many hospitals provide preceptors so that aspects of the situation can be pointed out and that during this stage of learning to set priorities based on salient aspects, no harm comes to the patients or to the new nurse.

Stage 3: Competent

Competence, typified by the nurse who has been on the job in the same or similar situations two to three years, develops when the nurse begins to see his or her actions in terms of long-range goals or plans of which he or she

25

is consciously aware. The plan dictates which attributes and aspects of the current and contemplated future situation are to be considered most important and those which can be ignored. Hence, for the competent nurse, a plan establishes a perspective, and the plan is based on considerable conscious, abstract, analytic contemplation of the problem. One preceptor describes her own evolution to the stage of competent, planned nursing from her earlier stimulus-response level of nursing:

I had four patients. One needed colostomy teaching, the others needed a lot of other things. When I went out there, instead of thinking before I went in the room . . . you get caught up . . . someone's I.V. stops, and you get caught up working on that. And then you forget to give someone their meds, and so you have to rush around and do that. And then someone is feeling nauseated and you try to make them feel better while they're sick. And then the colostomy bag falls off and you want to start teaching them. And all of a sudden the morning's gone and no one's gotten a bed bath.

Interviewer: So it would just be a reaction to the most urgent?

Nurse: I would just walk in there and get caught up with all their complaints, with no organization at all to what was going on. So now I come out of report and I know what their I.V.s are basically, and I have a couple of things that I know that I have to do. Before I go into the room, I write down what med I'm supposed to give for that day, and then I'll walk in there and make sure that everybody's I.V. is fine. You go from bed to bed and just say hi, just introduce yourself. But I give them the message that I'm just attending to business. I check their I.V.s, I check their dressings. And then I feel fine. I know they're not going to bleed to death; I know that their urine output is OK; I know that their

I.V.s are fine . . . then I have the whole morning set out and I can go ahead and do things. I am much more organized. I know what I have to do, and I arrange it with them and find out what they want to do.

The competent nurse lacks the speed and flexibility of the proficient nurse but does have a feeling of mastery and the ability to cope with and manage the many contingencies of clinical nursing. The conscious, deliberate planning that is characteristic of this skill level helps achieve efficiency and organization.

Implications for Teaching and Learning

There is a sophomoric quality to the competent stage. The clinical world seems organized, finally, after great effort. Nurses at this stage can benefit from decision-making games and simulations that give them practice in planning and coordinating multiple, complex patient care demands.

Stage 4: Proficient

Characteristically, the proficient performer perceives situations as wholes rather than in terms of aspects, and performance is guided by maxims. Perception is a key word here. The perspective is *not* thought out but "presents itself" based upon experience and recent events.

Proficient nurses understand a situation as a whole because they perceive its meaning in terms of long-term goals. An intensive care nursery clinician's description of neophyte nurses illustrates this change:

I think the biggest thing that's been on my mind for the last few weeks was whether I would be able to say at the end of the three-month period that the new graduate could give safe care, or does she just know how to manage the nursing care, or does she just know how to do specific tasks? To my mind, moving the child from Point A to Point B is what nursing is all about. You have to perform tasks along the way to make that happen, but performing the task isn't nursing . . . I wanted to see a light going on—that OK, here's *this* baby, this is where *this* baby is at, and here's where I want *this* baby to be in six weeks. What can I do today to make this baby go along the road to end up being better? It's that kind of thing that's just happening now. They're just starting to see the whole thing as a picture and not as a list of tasks to do.

The proficient nurse learns from experience what typical events to expect in a given situation and how plans need to be modified in response to these events. This is a web of perspectives and, as Stuart Dreyfus (1982) notes:

Except in unusual circumstances, the performer will be experiencing his current situation as similar to some brain-stored, experience-created, typical situation (complete with its saliences) due to recent past history of events . . . Hence the person will experience his or her situations at all times through a perspective, but rather than consciously calculating this perspective or plan, it will simply present itself to him or her. (p. 19)

Because of this experience-based ability to recognize whole situations, the proficient nurse can now recognize when the expected normal picture does not materialize. This holistic understanding improves the proficient nurse's decision making; it becomes less labored because the nurse now has a perspective on which of the many existing attributes and aspects present are the important ones. Whereas the competent person does not yet have enough experience to recognize a situation in terms of an overall picture or in terms of which aspects are most salient, most important, the proficient performer considers fewer options and hones in on an accurate region of the problem.

Aspects stand out to the proficient nurse as being more or less important to the situation at hand. The expert nurse, in talking about the patient's readiness to learn about his ileostomy (see pp. 79–80), said that she was glad she was able to stop everything and spend time with the patient at the precise moment when he was most ready to learn, and one can speculate that postponement would have been as unfortunate as a premature attempt to teach.

The proficient nurse uses maxims as guide(s), but a deep understanding of the situation is required before a maxim can be used. Maxims reflect what would appear to the competent or novice performer as unintelligible nuances of the situation; they can mean one thing at one time and quite another thing later. Once one has a deep understanding of the situation, however, the maxim provides direction as to what must be taken into consideration. Maxims reflect nuances of the situation. This is evident in the following account of weaning patients from a respirator:

Well, you look at their vital signs to see if there is anything significant . . . But even here you need to do a little guessing, in terms of whether the patient is just anxious because he's so used to the machine breathing for him . . . If they get a little anxious, you don't really want to medicate them, because you are afraid they will quit breathing, but on the other hand they may really need to calm down a bit, so it just depends on the situation. It is a real experiment. You have your groundwork, from what you have done in the past, and you know when you are going to get into trouble.

Implications for Teaching and Learning

Proficient performers are best taught by use of case studies where their ability to grasp the situation is solicited and taxed. Proficiency is enhanced if the student is required to cite experience and exemplars for perspective. Providing them with context-free principles and rules will only frustrate them and will usually stimulate them to give examples of situations where the principle or rule would be contradicted. At this point proficient performers can come to feel that the theory on which their skills and practices were initially based is a useless trapping. Or they may view the educator's elaborate decision analysis as the hard and unnecessarily elaborate way to solve a clinical problem that they can now grasp quickly by virtue of their experience. This will particularly be the case if the theory used is appropriate for teaching the beginner how to approach situations safely and is thus not appropriate for describing or explaining more complex or subtle aspects of the situation.

The proficient performer is best taught inductively, by beginning with a clinical situation and having the performer supply his or her ways of understanding the situation. When situations are introduced that exhaust the performer's way of understanding and approaching the situation, then a fruitful area of necessary learning has been uncovered. Learning exercises can be developed by having proficient clinicians supply two kinds of case studies from their own practice: (1) situations where they felt successful and thought their interventions made a difference; and (2) situations where they were not satisfied with their performance or felt in conflict about or confused by the situation. Case studies should contain some irrelevant, extraneous material and, in some instances, insufficient information to make an intelligent choice. To be effective, the case studies must have levels of complexity and ambiguity similar to real clinical situations.

It is the proficient performer who is most frequently able to recognize deterioration or patient problems prior to explicit changes in vital signs — that skill called the early warning signal (see pp. 100–102). Once proficient and expert nurse performers can be reliably identified, two practical questions can be addressed: What facilitates movement from the competent to proficient level other than time? What retards the movement?

Proficient performance can usually be found in nurses who have worked with similar patient populations for approximately three to five years. This time period is an estimate at this point and awaits further documentation. Proficient performance will regress to an analytic, competent level when novelty or the demand for an analytic, procedural description is required. The traditional expectation is that expert decisions are made by explicit evaluation of alternatives on the basis of comparison of salient elements. But in actuality, expert decisions are more holistic.

Stage 5: Expert

The expert performer no longer relies on an analytic principle (rule, guideline, maxim) to connect her or his understanding of the situation to an appropriate action.

31

The expert nurse, with an enormous background of experience, now has an intuitive grasp of each situation and zeroes in on the accurate region of the problem without wasteful consideration of a large range of unfruitful, alternative diagnoses and solutions.

Capturing the descriptions of expert performance is difficult, because the expert operates from a deep understanding of the total situation; the chess master, for instance, when asked why he or she made a particularly masterful move, will just say: "Because it felt right." "It looked good." Or when expert business decision makers are asked about which factors they would identify and what weights they would give them for a hypothetical decision, the most likely response would be, "Well, it all depends."

The problem that experts have in telling all they know is evident in the following excerpt from an interview with an expert psychiatric nurse clinician. She has worked in psychiatry for 15 years and is highly respected by both nurses and physicians for her clinical judgment and ability.

When I say to a doctor, "the patient is psychotic," I don't always know how to legitimize that statement. But I am never wrong. Because I know psychosis from inside out. And I feel that, and I know it, and I trust it. I don't care if nothing else is happening, I still really know that. It's like the feeling another nurse described in the small group interview today, when she said about the patient, "She just wasn't right." One of the things that I am doing now is getting some in-service in to talk to us about language. But all I am really trying to do is find words within the jargon to talk about something that I don't think is particularly describable.

The certainty in this brief excerpt should not be overgeneralized. This nurse is not saying that she never makes mistakes but instead is referring to her perceptual acuity – her recognitional ability. This kind of perceptual certainty does seem to come much like the well-documented ability to recognize the human face. This nurse is saying that she can recognize the changes common in psychosis because of her 15-year intensive study. And she is probably right. Her assertion opens up an interesting research question about whether this certainty is empirically borne out and, if so, which clinicians have it, and under what circumstances.

The nurse went on to describe a situation where she knew that a patient was being misdiagnosed as psychotic. She was convinced that the patient was only very angry; and the physician was equally convinced that the patient was psychotic and said, "We'll do an MMPI to see who's right." This nurse responded, "I am sure that I am right regardless of what the MMPI says." Fortunately for the nurse, the MMPI results backed up her assessment, because she had already begun a very successful intervention with the patient on the basis of her assessment.

Dreyfus and Dreyfus (1977) note:

> As long as the beginner pilot, language learner, chess player, or driver is following rules, his performance is halting, rigid, and mediocre. But with the mastery of the activity comes the transformation of the skill which is like the transformation that occurs when a blind person learns to use a cane. The beginner feels pressure in the palm of the hand which can be used to detect the presence of distant objects such as curbs. But with mastery the blind person no longer feels pressure in the palm of the hand, but simply feels the curb. The cane has become an extension of the body. (p. 12)

A similar transformation occurs with the expert nurse clinician's tools. As Dreyfus and Dreyfus (1977) describe the experienced performer:

The performer is no longer aware of features and rules, and his/her performance becomes fluid and flexible and highly proficient. The chess player develops a feel for the game; the language learner becomes fluent; the pilot stops feeling that he/she is flying the plane and simply feels that he/she is flying. (p. 12)

Now all this is not to say that the expert *never* uses analytic tools. Highly skilled analytic ability is necessary for those situations with which the nurse has had no previous experience. Analytic tools are also necessary for those times when the expert gets a wrong grasp of the situation and then finds that events and behaviors are not occurring as expected. When alternative perspectives are not available to the clinician, the only way out of a wrong grasp of the problem is by using analytic problem solving.

Implications for Teaching and Learning

Expert clinicians are not difficult to recognize because they frequently make clinical judgments or manage complex clinical situations in a truly remarkable way. But while recognition from colleagues and patients is apparent, expert performance may not be captured by the usual criteria for performance evaluation. It is at this juncture that the limits of formalism — that is, the inability to capture all the steps in the process of highly skilled human performance — become apparent (Benner, 1982, Kuhn, 1970, p. 192). To evaluate the expert level of performance an interpretive approach to describing nursing practice (see Chapter 3) and qualitative evaluation strategies must be added to the usual standards of practice or quantitative measures. The context and meanings inherent in the clinical situations strongly influence the expert's performance; therefore, evaluation strategies that rely on context-free principles and elements cannot capture the knowledge embedded in the expert's actual practice.

Systematic documentation of expert clinical performance is a first step in clinical knowledge development, and expert clinicians can benefit from systematically recording and describing critical incidents from their practice that illustrate expertise or a breakdown in performance. As expert clinicians document their performance, new areas of clinical knowledge are made available for further study and development.

Expert clinicians can also provide consultation for other nurses. They can be particularly effective in making a case for further medical evaluation when they detect early clinical changes. Except in intensive care units, however, most nurses performing at the expert level have little oportunity to compare and develop consensus on their observations with other nurses. Therefore, systematic efforts at developing a consensus about descriptive language and comparable observations among expert nurses would further enhance their performance.

The study of proficient and expert performance should make it possible to describe expert nursing performance and the resultant patient outcomes. This knowledge can be used to further develop the scope of practice of nurses who wish to and are capable of achieving excellence.

The vision of "what is possible" is one of the characteristics that separate competent from proficient and expert performance. Not all nurses will be able to become experts. Descriptions of excellence from expert nurse clinicians, however, offer new clinical possibilities for competent nurses and may facilitate their movement to the proficient stage. When experts can describe clinical situations where their interventions made a difference, some of the knowledge embedded in their practice becomes visible. And with visibility, enhancement and recognition of expertise become possible.

| The Meaning of Experience

Experience, as the word is used here, does not refer to the mere passage of time or longevity. Rather, it is the refinement of preconceived notions and theory through encounters with many actual practical situations that add nuances or shades of differences to theory (Gadamer, 1970; Benner & Wrubel, 1982). Theory offers what can be made explicit and formalized, but clinical practice is always more complex and presents many more realities than can be captured by theory alone.

True, theory guides clinicians and enables them to ask the right questions; this can be illustrated by the kind of transformation in practice brought about by theories (e.g., theories about the grieving process and about death and dying, mother-child separation studies in pediatrics, and infant-parent bonding studies in obstetrics). However, any nurse experienced in working with these theories finds differences that the formal theory fails to express. It is this clinical dialogue with theory that makes refinements accessible or possible for the experienced nurse.

On the other hand, theory and research are generated from the practical world — that is, from the practices of the experts in a field. Only from the assumptions and expectations embedded in expert clinical practice are questions generated for scientific testing and theory building. As long as the practices of the experts in a field go unnoticed and undocumented, and as long as the development of clinical expertise is limited by short clinical careers, an essential link in theory development in nursing will be missing. A nurse who has dealt with many people acquires a rich basis on which to interpret new situations, but this multifaceted knowledge with its concrete referents cannot really be put into abstract principles or even explicit guidelines.

There is a leap, a discontinuity, between the competent level and the proficient and expert levels. If experts are made to attend to the particulars or to a formal model or rule, their performance actually deteriorates.

This view of skill acquisition does not mean, however, that the rules and formulas just move to the unconscious level or go underground. This argument has been made in Hubert Dreyfus' book, *What Computers Can't Do: The Limits of Artificial Intelligence* (1979).

To get a feel for this model of skill acquisition, think of any experience in learning a skill such as riding a bicycle, driving a car, learning a second language, or giving intravenous fluids. In the beginning, performance is halting and rigid, and one must pay attention to explicit instruction. Performance is rule governed. The traditional Western assumption is that with experience and mastery of a skill, beginning rules just become unconscious. But this claim flies in the face of all evidence of masterful performance and ignores the role of perception in skilled performance.

Hubert and Stuart Dreyfus (1977) reported some air force studies that demonstrated that only by dropping the rules can one become really proficient. They cite the example of undergraduate pilots who are taught to follow a fixed sequence of visual scanning of instruments and dials. The air force researchers found that the instructors who were issuing these rules could find errors in the visual displays much more quickly than the trainees. They wondered whether the instructors applied the rules more quickly and more accurately than the student pilots, so they checked their eye movements and found that the instructors weren't using the rules that they were instructing the trainees in at all! Furthermore, their deviation from the rules allowed the instructors to perform faster and better.

Thus, an important assumption of the Dreyfus model is that with experience and mastery the skill is transformed. And this change brings about improvement in the performance. And if one insists that expert pilots, for example, pay attention to rules and guidelines that they may have used when they were beginners, their performance actually deteriorates.

One implication of this model is that formal structural models, decision analysis, or process models cannot describe the advanced levels of clinical performance observable in actual practice. An interpretive approach to describing nursing practice is presented in Chapter 3 as a means of describing the holistic, rapid decision making exhibited by experts and as a means of capturing the context and meanings inherent in actual nursing practice. Educators and practitioners have grappled with the problem of adequately describing the scope and depth of nursing as it is actually practiced. A limitation of both nursing process and decision analysis is that the task difficulty, relative importance, relational aspects, and outcomes of the skilled practice are not adequately captured without including the context, intentions, and interpretations of the skilled practice.

3 | An Interpretive Approach to Identifying and Describing Clinical Knowledge

 The interpretive approach used in the AMICAE project and this extension of it is rooted in the work of Heidegger (1962) and Taylor (1971) and is presented as an alternative method for the social sciences by Rabinow and Sullivan (1979). With such an interpretive strategy, synthesis, rather than analysis, is used. This allows a manageable yet rich description of actual nursing practice.

This model of study resembles the interpretation of a text. A sentence, for example, cannot be understood by analyzing the words alone. Rather, one understands a sentence as part of a larger whole and interprets its meaning from the context in which it is found. Similarly, behavior can be seen as having potentially multiple rather than single meanings. To understand behavior, therefore, one must look at it in its larger context. Practical knowledge, particularly at the expert level, must be studied holistically.

This can be easily illustrated by pointing out that the meaning of a bed bath changes with changes in the health status of the patient. Early in a patient's illness, a bed bath may be an essential comfort measure. With increasing recovery, this same bed bath may mean the excessive fostering of dependence. Thus to understand specific meaning of any behavior (or nursing care measure), one must know the specific context, and knowing the context inherently limits the possible meanings of behavior into manageable and relevant wholes. Therefore, the interpretive approach always relies on the particular context of the situation — that is, the timing, meanings, intentions of the particular situation.

With an interpretive approach, the intentions and understanding of the participants are taken into consideration and seen as dependent on a shared world of meanings. For example, intentions and empathy are a personal expression of the participants in a situation. Once described, however, they are clear to those who share the same background meanings. That is, the participants can talk about them, and the interpreter who shares their knowledge and experience base can understand them.

An interpretive approach avoids the problem of endless lists of tasks, with no guidelines for determining which ones are most important (Benner, 1982; Benner & Benner, 1979). This is because, once the context of the actual situation is described, the number of possible interpretations or meanings is limited. Usually one or two "best" interpretations emerge because the meaning of the situation is maintained rather than stripped away to objectified, context-free traits or behaviors (Dreyfus, 1979).

The domains and competencies (with their exemplars) of skilled nursing practice that will be presented in Chapters 4–10 illustrate this situation-based interpretive approach to identifying and describing knowledge embedded in clinical practice — that hybrid of theory and experience. This approach differs from listing the elemental or enabling skills that educators teach students in their early educational experiences. In contrast, the exemplars given here will illustrate nursing performance that represents a complex of enabling skills. Only as we see the whole can we adequately appreciate the significance of the nurse's contributions to patient welfare. And only as we see the whole can we begin to base nursing theory and nursing research on a well-charted background of clinical knowledge.

Nurses accrue clinical knowledge over time and lose track of what they have learned. One of the side benefits of the small group interviews used in this study (see pp. 14–16) was that nurses began to recognize that their clinical judgments had become more refined and astute over time. Preceptors began to recognize that their difficulties and even frustration in trying to share their knowledge with newly graduated nurses stemmed from the fact that they were offering knowledge far too complicated to be presented in instructions and cautionary statements to the learner. Much of their clinical know-how could only be *demonstrated* as the particular situations arose.

The variety and exceptions in actual clinical practice elude textbook descriptions but gradually yield to the experienced nurse's fund of past similar and dissimilar situations. It is this demonstration that is so essential to the neophyte.

Not all the exemplars to be presented reflect a proficient or expert level of practice, but all reflect clinical knowledge. The reader is encouraged to look for those areas of practical knowledge that were described in Chapter 1: graded qualitative distinctions, evidence of connoisseurship; assumptions, expectations, and sets;

paradigm cases; maxims; and finally, skills developed as a result of ad hoc, unplanned delegation of responsibility by physicians or other members of the health care team. Any nurse can compare these exemplars with similar and dissimilar situations from her or his own practice; when disagreement, agreement, questions, refinement, or extension of the exemplars is encountered, it will be an indication a new area of clinical knowledge is being uncovered.

In contrast to the situation-based, interpretive approach, the linear nursing process model can actually obscure the knowledge embedded in actual clinical practice, because that model oversimplifies and necessarily leaves out the context and content of nursing transactions. Nursing is relational and therefore cannot be adequately described by strategies that leave out content, context, and function. Tanner (1983) points to other research that corroborates that the nurse or physician begins with an early hypothesis about the diagnosis — what is termed in the Dreyfus model as a rapid grasp of the correct region of the problem.

It is possible to describe expert practice (Kuhn, 1979, p. 192), but it is *not* possible to recapture from the experts in explicit, formal steps, the mental processes or all the elements that go into their expert recognitional capacity to make rapid patient assessments. This does not mean, however, that the accomplishments and characteristics of expert nurse performance cannot be observed and described in narrative, interpretive form.

To assume that it is possible to capture *all* the steps in nursing practice is to assume that nursing is procedural rather than holistic. For example, a rapid grasp of the most important aspects of a problem (i.e., salience) is evident in expert performance. Attempts may be made to model or make explicit all the elements that go into a nursing decision, but experts do not actually make decisions in this elemental, procedural way. They do not build up their conclusions, element by element; rather, they grasp the whole. Even when they try to give detailed accounts of the elements that went into their decisions, essential elements are left out.

As Gestalt psychologists have long pointed out, the sum is greater than the parts. Also, the qualitative distinctions that expert clinicians make on the basis of their experience with many similar and dissimilar clinical situations cannot be transmitted by precise written descriptions. They are hard to teach too — for instance, differences in touch or feel — because beginners not only lack experience with "touch" and "feel" but also need procedural protocols and analytic strategies. The expert always knows more than he or she can tell (Polanyi, 1962). The clinician's knowledge is embedded in perceptions rather than precepts.

Performance Measurements

Performance measurements can be only as productive and accurate as the competencies selected to be measured. Measurement techniques, no matter how refined, cannot overcome the limitations incurred in the identification of competencies to be measured. Pottinger (1979) has pointed out the limitations of two commonly used competency identification strategies: (1) expert consensus, and (2) job analysis.

Little is known about how to measure a person's ability to *recognize* or *look for* problems that ought to be solved or the ability to implement choices or strategies for problem resolution. Thus, on the AMICAE project, an effort was made to identify competencies evident in actual clinical practice—for example, abilities such as coping with high threat situations; stability under pressure; compassionate, safe care of helpless infants or comatose patients (or other patients unable to protect themselves or who demand a certain standard of care); "hot" problem finding and "hot" problem solving (i.e., problem solving in crisis or high time-demand situations); coping with the pain of another person; or caring for the dying. But more is known about measuring problem-solving (judgment) capabilities when problem solving is reduced to defining the problem and ordering alternatives. Other aspects of the problem-solving process such as problem finding and solution implementation are usually omitted.

Identifying Domains and Competencies

In the interviews, the nurses were asked to describe patient care episodes in narrative form with as much detail as possible, including their intentions and interpretations of the events as well as the chronology of the action and outcomes. The transcripts and field notes were studied, and 31 competencies emerged from the analysis. These were then classified into seven domains on the basis of similarity of function and intent. These seven domains were derived inductively from the competencies themselves. The strength of this method lies in identifying competencies from actual practice situations rather than having experts generate competencies from models or hypothetical situations.

The interview transcripts and field notes were read several times, with a systematic attempt to move from the parts and back to the whole; this provided a basis for examining incongruities between the interpretation of the parts and the whole.

The interpretations in the form of identified competencies were presented to the research team for consensual validation. Further consensual validation can be supplied by the reader, who is given sufficient detail in the exemplar to judge whether the competency described is actually depicted by the exemplar. Multiple exemplars for each competency allowed confidence in the interpretation and prevented the interpreter from putting too much weight on a single episode. One patient–nurse episode could contain more than one competency, thus yielding more than one exemplar for one narrative account of a patient–nurse interaction.

The advantages of this method of identifying nursing competencies are that: (1) actual performance demands, resources, and constraints are described rather than hypothetical ones; and (2) this method provides a rich description of nursing practice. The context of this performance is maintained, and thus the description is synthetic, or holistic, rather than elemental and procedural.

The seven domains (see box on page 46) were identified after the exemplars were interpreted as representative of a particular competency. The competencies within each domain, in no way intended as an exhaustive or even comprehensive list, are presented in the chapters about the specific domains. Note that an adequate description of the competency is dependent on the exemplars. Adequate exemplars allow recognition of similar clinical situations even though many of the objective features may be quite different. The focus is on the whole situation rather than on breaking it down into specific tasks, as is done in teaching the beginner.

Conclusions will be drawn on the commonalities observed in the exemplars. Readers are encouraged to engage in active dialogue with these exemplars by comparing them to their own practice.

Summary

A situation-based interpretive approach to describing nursing practice overcomes some of the problems of reductionism inherent in a task analysis approach where tasks are listed with no content or goals. And it overcomes the problem of global and overly general descriptions based on nursing process categories.

Domains of Nursing Practice

The Helping Role

The Teaching–Coaching Function

The Diagnostic and Patient-Monitoring Function

Effective Management of Rapidly Changing Situations

Administering and Monitoring Therapeutic Interventions and Regimens

Monitoring and Ensuring the Quality of Health Care Practices

Organizational and Work-Role Competencies

4 | The Helping Role

Patients look to nurses for different kinds of help than they expect or receive from other helping professionals. Help seeking and help receiving are two different issues. A person can receive help without asking for it and can ask for it without being able to receive it. Even "help" sometimes does not help; some individuals with a strong need for personal control may not be able to acknowledge that they need help or even that they are being helped.

Many of the nurses we interviewed seemed to be aware of the personal issues of receiving and seeking help. Sometimes they covered their help and concern for their patients with humor or an air of nonchalance. In all cases they took special care to limit the patient's sense of obligation and tried to establish a context of attentiveness that was central to being a "nurse" and not dependent upon a social contract or exchange on the patient's part.

This is not to say that all nurses were helpful or uniformly astute in their helping role. It was clear to them that they were more helpful to some patients than others, and they frequently acknowledged the advantage of having different nurses on a unit who could relate to different patients. Nevertheless, I found myself frankly surprised at the quality of caring I observed. In an individualistic age where power, status, and control are taken for granted as the basic motivating forces in human interactions, I was prepared to observe power plays; instead, I found nurses who were skilled in avoiding power plays with their patients.

In our technological age, human pain and dilemmas are easily reduced to "problems to be solved." We analytically separate mind and body — the psychosocial and the physical — for study and then find it difficult to recombine these components to achieve a holistic or total approach to the patient. The exemplars in the helping domain illustrate, however, that a holistic approach does exist in the practical context of a committed nurse–patient relationship. The situation and the relationship determine what is possible and what is holistic. The hallmark of expert human decision making is that the situation structures the approach so that the response is only as orderly as the situation demands (Dreyfus, 1979, pp. 256–71).

For study purposes it is useful to break situations down and analyze them, but in the practical world the expert human decision makers bring a deep background understanding to the situation, so that they can grasp the whole and attend to the most salient aspects. They do this by sharing in the meanings embedded in the situation. If our notion of science dictates that we ignore "meanings," then we are cut off from practical holism (Dreyfus, 1980; Benner, in press).

The exemplars in this chapter demonstrate practical holism, but they also demonstrate that the nurse's helping goes beyond narrow definitions of "therapeutic," wherein change is considered in terms of measurable improvement, in the relinquishment of untenable commitments or meanings, or in goal setting. The helping to be described here encompasses transformative changes in meanings and sometimes simply the courage to be with the patient, offering whatever comfort the situation allows. This kind of helping cannot easily be discussed in generalities. It is best illustrated by the nurse's presentation of local, specific situations.

As shown in the box on page 50, the helping role has been broken down into eight competencies as these emerged from analysis of the observations and interviews.

The Healing Relationship: Creating a Climate for and Establishing a Commitment to Healing

A number of the episodes in which nurses thought their interventions made a difference in patient progress gave evidence of a healing relationship established between the nurse and the patient. Several steps were evident in this relational process:

1. Mobilizing hope for the nurse as well as for the patient.
2. Finding an acceptable interpretation or understanding of the illness, pain, fear, anxiety, or other stressful emotion.
3. Assisting the patient to use social, emotional or spiritual support.

EXEMPLAR I

An expert clinician described taking care of a young woman hospitalized with an advanced breast cancer. The woman was the mother of a young child and lived

Domain: The Helping Role

The Healing Relationship: Creating a Climate for and Establishing a Commitment to Healing

Providing Comfort Measures and Preserving Personhood in the Face of Pain and Extreme Breakdown

Presencing: Being with a Patient

Maximizing the Patient's Participation and Control in His or Her Own Recovery

Interpreting Kinds of Pain and Selecting Appropriate Strategies for Pain Management and Control

Providing Comfort and Communication Through Touch

Providing Emotional and Informational Support to Patients' Families

Guiding a Patient Through Emotional and Developmental Change: Providing New Options, Closing Off Old Ones: Channeling, Teaching, Mediating

> Acting as a psychological and cultural mediator
>
> Using goals therapeutically
>
> Working to build and maintain a therapeutic community

in a communal family. She had tried alternative sources of healing for her breast cancer, and these strategies had failed. She was now emaciated and had an advanced growth and open wound on her chest.

Interviewer: When I hear you describe your interaction with and thoughts about this patient, I hear that you made a commitment to her. For example, when you went skiing you thought about her; you came back and you checked the nursing notes and went in to see her even though she was not assigned to you. When did that commitment to her happen?

Expert Nurse: The first day I met her.

Interviewer: Tell us a little about the first encounter.

Expert Nurse: The only other cancer I had seen like that was when I was a student nurse (more than 20 years ago). That came back to me very vividly when I walked into her room. And the first patient I had, died. I had the feeling that this patient had the possibility of a good quality of life, if—and I read her notes closely—she had radiation therapy and chemotherapy and a good diet, and so forth—that her life span could be 8–10 years. Or maybe she even had a chance for a complete cure. And that to me was a challenge—to work with somebody like that. To support her in changing her lifestyle to improve her health.

Summary Statement   The nurse then described her interactions with this patient over the course of the next few weeks. She learned the patient's interpretation of her illness and encouraged her to be more assertive by encouraging her to practice assertiveness with her (the nurse), other members of the health care team, and her

51

family. She helped the patient work through the problem of increasing the protein in her diet.

Eventually the patient decided to have traditional medical treatment, radiation, and chemotherapy, augmented by her own support systems as a result of this nurse's interventions. The hope and concrete strategies offered by the nurse, along with the latter's expert interpretive skills, enabled this young woman to choose a therapeutic regimen. Eventually, the patient left the hospital with a healed wound and a sense of hope and possibility. The nurse was a key person in mobilizing the young woman's hope and in enabling her to choose an effective treatment.

EXEMPLAR II

Expert Nurse: The patient was a 17-year-old male admitted post c-spine fracture. The patient presented to the ICU awake, alert, and quadriplegic. His vital signs were stable, his respirations shallow but apparently adequate. Within 24 hours, due to poor ventilatory effort, significant lung consolidation developed. The doctors decided to intubate him in order to provide positive airway pressure from a ventilator. Due to the instability of his fracture, other respiratory measures could not be undertaken.

The patient was extremely apprehensive about his intubation. His respiratory rate increased dramatically after the tube was passed. His respiratory rate increased into the 40s and his PCO_2 was dropping. The patient was unable to decrease his respiratory rate due to his high anxiety. Mild sedation was of no help. The doctors were considering increasing his sedation enough to knock out his respiratory drive so that we could totally control his ventilation with this respirator. This increased his anxiety even more. I knew the complications which could arise with this measure. It would have added to his already

monumental problems with recovery and rehabilitation—
something he didn't need. My question: Couldn't this be
avoided? I was impressed with the positive attitude and
emotional strength of this young man. I just *knew* we could
resolve this problem—his anxiety and thus rapid respiration
rate—without using such drastic measures. I began to talk with
him—reassuring him, using my calmest and most reassuring
voice. I spoke assuredly, honestly, professionally, and yet
personally. I intervened in his behalf with his multiple
physicians; I explained my "gut feeling," my concerns for his
recovery, and negotiated for more time to attempt to resolve this
problem.

He could not speak, as he was intubated. He could not write,
as he was quadriplegic, and we didn't allow him to nod his
head due to his unstable neck fracture. His only communication
was with his eyes and his amazing ability to mouth words
clearly and understandably.

It took three and half hours before he began to relax. He
needed to understand what had happened, and was presently
happening, to him. He needed to be reassured, and most of all
to learn to trust us. He needed to know what the future might
hold for him. He needed to know that we cared about *him*, as
an individual, not just another helpless patient. As he began to
comprehend all the others, he learned to trust us; that was the
key. He needed to be involved, not just prescribed to, and he
felt so very helpless.

This incident is critical to me because it was what nursing is
all about for me. In critical care nursing, these interactions are
few and far between. The point was made by one simple
statement he mouthed to me late in the day—when he had a
respiration rate in the 20s, and he was no longer threatened
with having the few remaining functional muscles chemically
paralyzed. His words were: "Thank you. You've really helped
me a lot. I don't want to imagine what would have happened to
me if you weren't here and hadn't cared."

Interviewer: What were your thoughts, your concerns,
during this time?

Expert Nurse: My concerns were that I could be wrong, and that I was causing him undue stress and prolonged high level of CO_2, and that he would not respond. I was thinking: "Learn to be a fighter right from the start. You have a very long fight ahead. Don't give in. If only I can gain your trust. I don't want you to become less than a person—a sedated, controlled physiological state. Please relax, relax." I felt a sense of urgency, as his respiratory rate had to come down. I felt pity for him. I felt a need to succeed. I was sad—he was so young and vital, and his normal youth was snatched away. I wanted him to have every chance. After the incident I was elated. I felt fulfilled and proud. The most demanding part of the incident was the frustration. Needing to remain patient—to keep an even temperament while repeating phrases for the umpteenth time.

Summary Statement This nurse used her judgment that the patient could regain control over his respirations and that such an accomplishment was important to his morale and even to his recovery. Even so, as she makes clear, she could not be sure that her intervention would be successful. Success was clear only after nearly four hours of constant reassurance and encouragement of the patient.

In both this exemplar and the previous one, the nurse mobilizes her own hope as well as that of the patients; finds an interpretation or understanding of the situation acceptable to them; and helps them use their own support systems. In the second exemplar, the nurse says that she was "impressed with the positive attitude and emotional strength of the young man." She recognized that the patient was feeling helpless and would feel even more helpless if he lost control over his respirations. In the first exemplar the nurse helped the patient draw on her own support systems and alternative ways of healing while incorporating new strategies. In each case, the nurse's interventions came from a committed, involved stance rather than a detached one. The involved stance seems to be a hallmark of the nurse's helping role.

Providing Comfort Measures and Preserving Personhood in the Face of Pain and Extreme Breakdown

Many nurses must face the fact that there is little they or others can do to prolong the life of a patient. On the other hand, there is often some room to enhance the quality of life, short though it may be, of the patient's last days in the hospital. While the nurse must be able to give up on trying to save a patient's life, she or he must not avoid the patient and must still find ways of providing comfort for him and his family.

EXEMPLAR I

An expert nurse described how she and others attended a dying elderly patient on the ICU unit.

Expert Nurse: We had an 86-year-old woman who has had chronic obstructive pulmonary disease for many, many years. She has had lots of supportive treatment, with oxygen treatments, and a lot of supportive assistance medically. The son has been very close to her and has spent a lot of time in caring for her. She was readmitted to our unit last week, very ill, and the son talked with the physician and made the decision that we would not give her any more medical support, that we would just make her comfortable, and let her die on her own.

She was my patient. And you know just because they are not going to do anything else for her doesn't mean that I stop caring for her. So I gave her her bath. She had her little suitcase there with all her little things. I have known her for a while. She is very meticulous and very neat. So I put her in one of her gowns and propped her up all around in her bed with pillows. I didn't feel that I was doing anything special for her. But the son told me at the end how much it meant to him to see that the nurses still cared for his mother.

EXEMPLAR II

An expert nurse describes caring for a diabetic patient who is blind and gravely ill.

Expert Nurse: And that day we washed her hair which hadn't been washed in weeks. We got her up out of bed and sat her up. She just loved that, to get up off her back. She had been so sick and forced to be on her back; she had a decubitus forming. Any *little* thing that we did for her—wash her hair, set her up, take her limbs through a range of motion—was just a delight for her. And she let us know that. She just told me how wonderful it was to have people read to her, so I did bring a book in. She had told me about a book she was interested in, and her cousin, who was a student nurse here, and I would take turns reading to her. And she just loved that.

Summary Statement   In both exemplars, the patient's personhood is attended to by the nurse. This means that the nurse must be able to overcome the usual mind set of "doing for" and "curing" the patient, and instead contribute to and facilitate the patient's sense of personhood, meaning, and dignity.

| Presencing: Being with a Patient

Nurses are often trained to believe that they are most effective when *doing for* a patient. Several nurses noted, however, the essential importance of just *being with* a patient:

EXEMPLAR I

Expert Nurse: It is a person-to-person kind of thing, just being *with* somebody, *really* communicating with people. And sometimes I just feel a closeness. You talk about empathy or whatever, but somebody is frightened and just sitting down and listening to people, it's not that you even have to say anything. And I think that is an important thing, because I tend to always want to have an answer. But when I have just kept my mouth shut and just listened, it's been much more effective; just the fact that somebody is *there* just to *listen* to somebody express their concerns, and that you don't necessarily have to have an answer or a suggestion or solve the problem, but just because they've been able to have someplace to talk about it. It makes it easier.

EXEMPLAR II

Participant Observation of an Expert Nurse: Elizabeth, an expert nurse, cared for a patient who went into septic shock and experienced extreme chills. Once the situation was under control and there was nothing else to do, Elizabeth held the patient by his shoulders very tightly, simply being with him through the coldness of his moments. It seemed her simply being there provided comfort for the patient.

EXEMPLAR III

Expert Nurse: We had a woman who came in with diagnosis of diverticulosis. She had had bilateral mastectomies, and on her laparotomy they found her belly full of cancer. Her surgery was open-and-close. The attending told her husband and instructed him not to tell his wife until she had recovered from her surgery. Her prognosis was grave, probably only a few weeks. The day I remember is when she was very close to death and we were all waiting for her son to arrive from Texas. He hadn't seen his mother in several years, but his mother very much wanted to see him before she died. She was delirious and her husband was frantic with anxiety that his son wouldn't arrive in time. I spent much of that time with him in her room talking to them both and bathing her. She was incontinent and bleeding from many orifices. We then heard that the plane her son was on was two hours late, which heightened everyone's anxiety. He [the son] finally arrived and I told him what to expect when he entered the room. They spent 15 minutes together, the three of them, before she died. She was alert and talking the whole time. We all cried that day, amazed and reaffirmed by this example of human strength.

Summary Statement   The expert nurses here had the self-esteem and self-confidence to see the value of their presence for their patients. They point to the importance of touch and person-to-person contact between patient and nurse. They also speak to nurses' need to allow patients to ventilate their feelings, often without speaking at all themselves.

Maximizing the Patient's Participation and Control in His or Her Own Recovery

This competency entails at least two components: sensing a patient's strength, drive, desire, and ability to improve, and mobilizing these forces in the relationship between the nurse and the patient. In some

cases it may also entail serving as a patient advocate —
i.e., arguing against a potentially harmful technological
intervention in favor of the patient's ability to control
and improve his condition without the intervention. In
some cases it is a matter of negotiating for more time.

In situations like these, nurses used their relationship with the patient to elicit patients' own involvement and control. Behind this competency is a
determined effort to maximize the patient's control
over his life.

EXEMPLAR I

An experienced nurse described several episodes with
an elderly patient who was recovering from a mild
stroke. The patient, a concert pianist, was depressed
over the weakness in her right hand. The first incident
described was in response to the patient's refusal to go
to physical therapy.

Expert Nurse: I just sat down and listened and talked to
her. I did not say that I wanted her to go to physical therapy, but
that was my intention. I said to her that she was showing some
progress. "Think about two days ago; today you can move your
fingers a little bit more. You have made progress because of the
exercise. If you keep doing these exercises, I expect that you
will be able to have more use of your hands." I encouraged
her — pointing out the positive things because she was only
zeroing in on the negative things and looking at how much she
didn't have. I reminded her that when she first came in that her
arm was weak and that she needed a lot of help to eat. Now she
is able to hold a cup by herself. Now she is able to move her
fingers and raise her arm; she could even raise it over her head.
I said, "Look, you couldn't do that yesterday and you are able to

do that today." I just went through all the things that I could see that I hadn't seen the day before. After our talk she went to physical therapy.

Over time the expert nurse continued to provide feedback on the patient's progress and provide a perspective on the amount of time required for recovery and the comparative mildness of the patient's current limitations and possibility for recovery and ability to teach piano again. The patient wanted to keep as many of her former activities as possible. The nurse had her daughter bring in a small practice keyboard that the patient could use in the hospital. The nurse, the patient, and the daughter planned ways of providing periods of rest and limiting stair climbing at home so she could continue to teach piano students.

EXEMPLAR II

The patient was a 36-year-old man who had a history of multiple surgeries and complications. He had a history of ulcers and came as a transfer from another hospital after having surgery for hemorrhagic pancreatitis. He ended up with another surgery from which he emerged minus most of his pancreas and with multiple tubes, a huge abdominal wound, several I.V.s, etc. He was a person who had always been independent and was having an extremely hard time coping with being ill and helpless. He went up and down in his postop course, but finally reached a point where he was so angry and so depressed that he refused any further treatments, procedures, and blood work. He also refused to ambulate or do much of his self-care.

We had a pretty close relationship by that time so I went in to talk to him. He told me, "I'm so sick of being poked all the time, and not having any say in any of this. I'm so helpless. People are constantly doing things to me!" I told him that while the circumstances would be hard to change (given his condition and his need for hospitalization), he could shift his point of view. I told him that he did have a choice in all of this (in fact, he had already chosen) by coming to a different hospital for better care. And that instead of seeing himself as having things being done *to* him, he could view it as things being done *for* him to help him get better. I told him that while he felt helpless about what we were doing to him physically, he was the only one who could help himself mentally by keeping this whole thing in perspective. . . that he needed to remember that he was a *person*. . . that he was more than this sickness he was going through. He was very quiet during my talk and I couldn't really tell if I was getting through. I felt at times like I might be expecting too much from him, but I told him as his friend I felt obligated to tell him the way I felt.

The next morning when I came to work, I saw him sitting out in the hall by the window laughing and smiling. When I asked him what had changed for him, he said, "You were right! I'm just going to choose to be here and let all of you help me get well as fast as I can!"

I really felt like I made a difference in this man's life in helping him cope with circumstances he thought were beyond his control, just by helping him tap into inner strengths.

Summary Statement In both exemplars the nurse helps the patient regain a sense of control and active participation in recovery. Many patients feel alienated from their recovery and treatment; frequently it is the nurse who assists the patient in regaining a sense of participation and control.

Interpreting Kinds of Pain and Selecting Appropriate Strategies for Pain Management and Control

Pain management and control have become more sophisticated and specialized in terms of varying the pain control and management procedures to meet particular kinds of pain. Selecting the appropriate strategy at the right time falls into the domain of nursing judgment as illustrated in the exemplar below:

EXEMPLAR

Expert Psychiatric Nurse: I was called to the emergency room to do a crisis intervention. The medical doctor said that the patient is hysterical, complains of severe back pain, and he thought the patient was a psychiatric case. I saw the young man and recognized that he was truly in a lot of pain. He had fallen 15 feet several months ago. There was a pending disability case. He was hysterical, in part, because he was not being believed, and also probably because of the pressure of the pending court case. I think it was twofold. I thought that admitting him to a psychiatric unit was not an appropriate intervention. Being labeled a psychiatric case would also make his court case look less believable. I also believed that someone in that amount of pain should not be on the psychiatric unit. If he was going to be admitted, he would have to be admitted to the medical unit for further evaluation. I was able to get a shot of Demerol, which helped. His body was full of spasms. The next crisis intervention person also agreed with my decision, and the patient subsequently went home. Patients who are in a lot of pain will get hysterical, especially when they are not believed. I felt really good about that decision.

Providing Comfort and Communication Through Touch

Nurses frequently use touch to provide comfort and reach out to a withdrawn, depressed patient. Often, this human and warm contact is the only avenue of comfort and communication available.

EXEMPLAR I

Participant Observation: Elizabeth went and washed her hands, got some cream from the man's drawer. She helped him remove his pajama top and sat down on the bed next to him. He sat on the end of the bed, looking rather gloomy and uncommunicative. Elizabeth put a lot of cream on her hands and warned him that it was going to be cold—apologizing for it. For a while she used both hands while massaging him. At other times she used her right hand, rubbing him firmly, but obviously gently. There was not too much conversation at this time. Elizabeth said that she wished she could do it longer, but did make it rather short, I thought, compared to what I had seen her do before with a patient when the unit was less busy. When she was done, she took a washcloth and rubbed his back clean of the cream. She told him they would try to give him another one later on. In the hall, I asked Elizabeth about this transaction. First, was this routine with him? Yes, she said. He's been having trouble with his back; he has lower back pain. I asked what was wrong with him. He's had a section of his colon removed and now has a colostomy, she said. "They found a lot of cancer, and he's in pretty bad shape, but he doesn't talk about his feelings much. I like to use the back rub as a chance to talk to him and as a different way of communicating with him."

63

EXEMPLAR II

Expert Nurse: It was an emergency situation. A patient was having many things done to her. She was being intubated and such. In the midst of it, when she needed someone, we were the only ones there to hold her hand. She was in tears. She didn't know what was happening. She was deaf, but she *knew* it was serious; she was crying—you'd see the tears coming down her face. The physicians were trying to intubate her, and Ann, the other nurse, and I would just sit there between all the vitals and stuff. We would hold her hand and say, "Everything is under control." You just felt that was one of the most important things to do. Because she *needed* someone and she could only receive comfort and caring through touch and sight.

Summary Statement   Nurses have traditionally been the ones to use touch therapeutically. Touch conveys relational and support messages as well as physical stimulation and comfort. It is perhaps symbolic of the direct laying on of hands, so central to nursing care. But touch, like any other form of communication, has many messages and must be used with discretion.

Providing Emotional and Informational Support to Patients' Families

The nurses provided many examples of considering the patient's family as their clients and as important resources for the patient's recovery. They often provided emotional support to the families or gave them the opportunity and the information necessary for them to provide physical care for the patient. Thus, the nurse supports and maximizes the family members' positive role in the patient's recovery, as well as providing them with emotional and informational support.

EXEMPLAR I

Expert Nurse: We had a patient who had a ruptured aneurysm and he was really, really critical. They didn't think he was going to make it at all. And the wife had no family member, no support from anybody. There was only she and her husband. They had no children. And I was able to be with her. I took her down to lunch and when she was here I always made her feel like she could find out how her husband was doing. In a lot of intensive care units, visitors are hands off, and that's true for visitor visitors, but for the immediate family, I'm really of the philosophy that it's good for the patient and it's good for the family if they can be with the patient more. And it was just really important for her to be able to be there with her husband. So I'd do what I could for her and let her come in and just sit there by the bed. That's all she wanted to do. And then I would talk to her. I would answer any questions that she had and explain to her what we were doing. He ended up having to be dialyzed. I was always able to explain things to her. She called me at home a couple of times. That makes me feel real good when I can do that. And then when he went home, he did get much better.

EXEMPLAR II

Expert Nurse: And so I stayed with the patient in labor, and it had been three hours and there hadn't been any change. I felt as though I didn't want to even say anything to her. She was so uncomfortable. She'd already had some medication, and she wanted desperately to be progressing, and she wasn't. Her husband was very supportive and he really wanted to be taking care of his wife. When I helped her up to the restroom, he wanted to do that. So I took the I.V. off and unhooked her from the IVAC and took those. And rather than me telling her that she was doing a very good job of her breathing and her relaxing, he really wanted to be the coach, so I let him. Because after a couple of times I sort of caught on that this was what he was doing, and that he was doing a very good job. And it was what he needed to be doing. So I let him do that. In the meantime, the doctor calls and wants to know what she's doing. Well, she hadn't made any progress, but she's having good labor. And he said, "Well, let's give her another hour." But it turned out that she did not make any progress and had to have a Caesarian section. . . The doctor calls up and says, "We're going to do her right now." Well, I talked to him about doing it in the delivery room so her husband could be present, because husbands aren't permitted in the operating room. In addition, she wanted to be awake, so I tried to find an anesthesiologist who would go along with that. It worked out well. The husband was able to be with his wife, and to take pictures.

Summary Statement   In both these exemplars, the nurse considers the family member's needs as well as the patient's. The nurse must know when to move aside and allow family members a greater role in the care of the patient and when to relieve the family member.

Guiding Patients Through Emotional and Developmental Change: Providing New Options, Closing Off Old Ones: Channeling, Teaching, Mediating

The psychiatric nurse has unique functions in the acute hospital by virtue of the nature of psychatric illness and the context of the psychiatric unit. While most nurses use their knowledge of psychiatric nursing in almost every patient situation, the competencies listed in this domain were generated from an acute in-hospital psychiatric setting. What sets the competencies apart from the others are the particular kinds of therapeutic goals and intentions of the psychiatric nurse.

The psychiatric nurse uses many ways to channel a patient into ways of being that hold more potential for growth. As a guide and mediator helping confused people carve a path into a more shared, less idiosyncratic world, the nurse is firm, direct, and approaches the patient with as much clarity as possible. In trying to help people change, the nurse (1) acts as a psychological and cultural mediator; (2) uses goals therapeutically; and (3) works to build and maintain a therapeutic community.

Psychological and Cultural Mediator

Psychiatric patients are often outsiders; they do not feel and see things in the same way that "normal" people see and feel things, and many of the taken-for-granted rules and meanings of other people do not hold for them. Thus, the psychiatric nurse *mediates* between the patient and the other, more normal culture. She learns to understand patients in their particularity; she understands their particular language and the feelings behind their behavior and words; she learns to understand the private and idiosyncratic meanings that things might have for them.

The nurse learns to understand and remember what patients do not understand — what cannot be taken for granted when interacting with them. She learns to "read" particular patients — e.g., to assess and distinguish different levels of regression in order to know what kind of language to use — and also knows whether a patient is in danger. Finally, the nurse needs to learn the patterns and scenarios of patients in order to anticipate a patient's response to something.

At the base of this understanding is an openness and acceptance of the "otherness" of the patient. Sometimes nurses get a head start on this understanding through personal experience of their own and through frequent experiences with patients with a particular problem.

EXEMPLAR I

Expert Psychiatric Nurse: I was making my rounds. And I walked in and I said, "Hi, I'm Sue. You must be Ann." And she said, "What the hell is it to you? I'm so goddamned mad." I was just amused by it and said, "Well, why don't you tell me about it?" I knew from the beginning that there was such pain under her vile language—such intensity, almost agony. And I didn't even know her history. I didn't know anything about her. But I knew that. And over the next month I found out about the agony and the pain.

Sometimes the experiences of a patient are extremely foreign to the nurse. In this case understanding comes by letting patients "teach the nurse what it is like to be in their shoes."

EXEMPLAR II

An expert psychiatric nurse tells what she learned from a cerebral palsy patient.

Expert Nurse: She taught me about what it's like to be trapped in a body that won't do what you want it to do. She taught me what it was like to have people look at you and treat you as if you were retarded, even though your mind is fine, but because your jaw is slack or your speech is different or your gait is funny or your arm flies around, you get treated as if your mind is also impaired. She taught me what it was like to spend so much time and energy trying to control your body that you don't have a whole lot of energy left for anything else.

While the psychiatric nurse is trying to understand the meanings of the patient, he or she is also trying to teach the patient about the world of ordinary people and working in different ways to create a common, shared culture on the unit or in a group in which everyone can participate. The nurse does this by translating for patients what their behavior means to other people and also explains the patient to the members of the group or community, so they can understand and not ostracize the patient for the behavior.

For example, a nurse tells a patient, "People will get angry when you talk to them like that," and also explains what other people will or will not do. Nurses do this by clearly stating their expectations, by setting goals, by establishing and implementing rules and contracts that people must obey, and then helping them achieve them.

The nurse gives patients a language in which they can express their feelings in ways that other people can understand and won't find threatening. In these and other ways, the psychiatric nurse can be seen as a psychological and cultural mediator for patients, helping them become more social and cultural beings who can interact more satisfyingly with other people.

The nurse's mediating and facilitating role will depend on the particular stance that she takes vis-a-vis the patient — one that separates nurse from patient but is still supportive. The nurse is *with* the patient without fusing her own boundaries, selfhood, or integrity. Nurses are not endangered by the patient's perceptions or behavior.

Second, the patient's ultimate success (behavioral or symptomatic improvement, recovery, etc.) is not for the nurse's benefit or reputation; its intrinsic worth is to the patient. In other words, the nurse is on the patient's side for the patient's benefit, not to gain personal gratification in dependent relationships or a sense of aggrandizement based upon the patient's success. Since the disturbed patient's ego boundaries are so fragile, this position on the part of the nurse often reduces the patient's stress or tension and frees him to explore new possibilities. The patient no longer has to resist the therapist in order to gain self-definition.

There are many ways in which one sees this stance in operation. For example, the nurse does not accept responsibilty for the patient, but rather deflects it back to the patient. The responsibility for the patient's life belongs to the patient, and so do any claims of success. It may be difficult to do, but the psychiatric nurse gives the patient's life back to him or her.

EXEMPLAR III

Expert Psychiatric Nurse (talking to interviewer):   And I think putting that out clearly to the patient, that is to say, my expectation for you is that you take care of yourself and that you don't ask me to take care of you. I'm not responsible for you. I have a full-time job being responsible for me, and once you start being responsible for you, that will be a full-time thing also. That can be delivered with a lot of caring and it can be delivered with a lot of support, but I think it must be delivered. . .

Summary Statement Mediating psychological and cultural meanings is a broad competency that takes time to develop as nurses must refine their ability to develop therapeutic relationships and interpret a broad range of unusual and normal meanings and behavior.

Using Goals Therapeutically

The nurse understands the usefulness of goals in establishing a commitment to therapy and in maintaining the commitment to work toward wellness over a long period. These goals have to be realistic and workable for the individual and must aim toward improved social and psychological functioning. And the nurse must help the patient to recognize when he or she has been successful.

This skill differs from "making an assessment of the patient's potential for wellness and potential for responding to various treatment procedures" (to be discussed later), in that such intervention is possible only after the nurse has accurately made such an assessment. Using goals therapeutically requires that the nurse select the appropriate level of goals at the appropriate time in the patient's progress.

EXEMPLAR

Expert Psychiatric Nurse: (description of a patient in group therapy) She re-established contact with her children after not

71

seeing them for a long time and she now has a really healthy thing going on with them in which she sees them every other weekend. She brings them home with her. She is answering their questions about why mommy can't be with them all the time. And she's answering them honestly. "It's not because you're bad kids, and it's not because you're asking too much. It's because I can't do it, but that doesn't mean I don't love you, and it doesn't mean I don't want to see you and it doesn't mean I'm not going to be involved in your life." She's doing that in such a responsible way. And I'm really proud of her.

Last year she had her first paid vacation of her entire life because she was a member of the working force and had had a job long enough to actually earn a vacation. That was absolutely a highlight for her. I mean, it sounds so simple, but one of the things that we really address in the group is that if you want to feel good about yourself, you have to do the kinds of things that can help you feel good. You know, people don't feel good when they're sitting back being taken care of by other people or an institution like welfare or whatever. And if you want to feel good, then you're probably going to have to take the steps that it takes to get better feelings. That sounds so straightforward and so obvious, yet it is almost never addressed by a psychiatrist. I don't know that I've ever heard of it being addressed in all the years I've been on the unit. And that is, if you want to feel better about yourself, you have to do reasonable things to feel better. And being a responsible citizen is one of them. We really stress responsibility. And that means fully responsible. If you can't do it, it's OK. Own that. Own that you can't do it, and then if it's something that needs to be done—like your children being taken care of or whatever—then you get that done by someone who can do it.

Summary Statement In the exemplar, the nurse describes the very practical and realistic goals that the patient aimed for and achieved. She was not able to have her children with her all the time, and she could be honest with them about her limitations. Her ability to do this is a major achievement. The nurse recognizes this, and her pride in her patient's achievement helps the patient see her own improvement and accomplishment. The paid vacation is another such achievement. Both her ability to find a way to be with her children and her holding onto her job are successes in the area of social functioning that could have resulted from improved psychological functioning, but also feed back to the latter area: the woman has been helped to feel better about herself.

Building and Maintaining a Therapeutic Community

Patients interpret the meaning of psychiatric events — such as "acting out," suicide, adverse drug reactions, being discharged, getting well — in terms of their own ability to get well, control themselves, and in terms of the staff's ability to assist them, protect them from injury, and help them get well. Thus the nurse and other psychiatric team members must attend to the meanings likely to be felt and understood by other patients when notable changes occur within the psychiatric community. This means that the nurse must assess patients' interpretations of psychiatric events and attempt to reinterpret or reshape the meaning of the event if the meaning is disruptive to the therapeutic goals (i.e., hope, trust, confidence) of the therapeutic community.

The therapeutic community also provides a microcosm of a social system, a network of relationships, an arena for working out the issues of trust, conflict, and cooperation. Thus the community is a basic therapeutic tool and, as such, must be built, monitored, and maintained. As one nurse stated: "Things that happen on the unit are experienced personally. For example, if a patient is discharged who is saying, 'I'm not ready to go,' or if a patient is transferred to a locked unit, or is restrained or attempts suicide, the other patients wonder: Will you discharge me prematurely . . . or transfer me . . . or restrain me . . . ?"

EXEMPLAR

Expert Psychiatric Nurse: An unusual day that stands out for me was a day in which a patient had suicided on the unit [during the night], and the psychiatrist did not come in. We notified the family. We gave the night staff an option of staying over for the community meeting of the patients — got the patients up for breakfast, then called this special meeting to inform them of the incident and allow them to talk about how they were feeling. We wanted to deal with and respond to feelings that this loss brought up, e.g., "Why didn't you protect him? — Can you protect me?" Because a suicide brings up panic and brings down impulse control on the unit, we worked with patients to devise a special three-day emergency plan, whereby we intensified one-to-one availability, stopped off-unit privileges, stopped passes unless plans were detailed with a resource nurse, and stopped admissions temporarily.

Summary Statement The nurse as well as other members of the therapeutic community has a responsibility for and becomes skilled in building and maintaining a therapeutic community. Frequently this entails interpreting events on the unit to the patients in situations where misinterpretation or misunderstanding might occur. It also entails building and maintaining relationships with other members of the therapeutic community to create an atmosphere of trust and shared communication.

| Summary and Conclusions

The research and practical implications of this and the other domains will be discussed more fully in Chapter 11 and the implications for career development and education will be discussed in Chapter 12. The most significant implications must be left to practicing clinicians who examine these exemplars in the context of their own practices. There are distinct barriers and limitations to making standards of these exemplars, because they cannot be quantified nor legislated; they come from a committed, involved, nurse–patient relationship. Although commitment cannot be legislated, it *can* be facilitated and rewarded.

The exemplars in this chapter challenge nurses to extend their helping powers so that the restoration and empowerment of patients receive as much emphasis as technical care. This requires expertise in listening and in understanding what an illness means to the patient, what it interrupts, and what recovery means. These exemplars challenge nurses to have lines of help available that are as specific and unique as the situation itself. They challenge nurses to take risks for the patient's sake. But most of all they challenge nurses to own their own unique helping role. Nurses will not become more powerful or gain more status by ignoring their unique contributions simply because they are not easily replicated, standardized, or interpreted.

5 | The Teaching–Coaching Function

    Nurses have long recognized how significant teaching is to the patient's preparation for and recovery from surgery. Nurses provide benchmarks and timetables to the hospitalized patient who does not know what to expect during the course of an illness. But the hospital environment is not the only novel, foreign part of an acute illness. The illness itself replaces familiar bodily responses with unfamiliar ones and, correctly or not, patients interpret these responses; sometimes they mistake a sign of improvement for a sign of deterioration. So nurses, when possible, forewarn them what to expect, correct misinterpretations, and offer explanations for the bodily changes. Doctors are perceived to be too busy to talk about the minutiae of symptoms, even though the latter may occupy a great deal of the patients' thoughts. Patients frequently check out their questions with the nurse before asking the doctor. Thus, nurses become experts in coaching a patient through an illness. They take what is foreign and fearful to the patient and make it familiar and thus less frightening.

Teaching and learning transactions require great skill under the best of circumstances, but they take on new demands and require different skills when the learner is threatened and ill. Expert nurses have learned to communicate and to teach in extreme situations. And in this teaching they are forced to use themselves, their attitudes, tone of voice, humor, skill, and a variety of approaches to the patient.

We have much to learn from the uncharted wisdom of the nurse who is an expert teacher and coach. But learning from experts requires attention to the context and to the avoidance of hasty generalizations. For example, sometimes the coach must be stern and "take over" for the patient who is experiencing panic. Later, that same nurse will have to encourage the patient to take over. Self-care is highly valued but to expect it in the extremes of a serious illness is often unrealistic.

The variability in the demands, resources, and constraints of the situation militate against context-free generalizations. Therefore, much of the skill embedded in expert teaching–coaching will be missed if we study only the formal, planned teaching–learning sessions. We need also to study the teaching and coaching that is embedded in skilled nursing care. We will be oversimplifying this role if we look only for information giving or formal "precepts" taught, because the more significant learning lies in coping with illness and mobilizing for recovery. These expert nurses not only offer information, they offer ways of being, ways of coping, and even new possibilities for the patient by means of the perspectives and the practices that are embedded in good nursing care. Their competencies are listed in the box on page 79.

Domain: The Teaching–Coaching Function

> Timing: Capturing a Patient's Readiness to Learn
>
> Assisting Patients to Integrate the Implications of Illness and Recovery into Their Lifestyles
>
> Eliciting and Understanding the Patient's Interpretation of His or Her Illness
>
> Providing an Interpretation of the Patient's Condition and Giving a Rationale for Procedures
>
> The Coaching Function: Making Culturally Avoided Aspects of an Illness Approachable and Understandable

Timing: Capturing a Patient's Readiness to Learn

Although many nursing activities are dictated by a regular schedule, discretion is sometimes essential in the timing of an intervention. Assessing where a patient is, how open he is to information, deciding when to go ahead even when the patient does not appear ready, are key aspects of effective patient teaching.

EXEMPLAR

Expert Nurse: I had a very satisfying teaching experience with a patient today because I was able to stop everything and

79

spend an hour and a half with him, teaching him at the precise moment that he was most ready to learn. It was a tough decision, because it entailed stopping all other responsibilities and telling everybody that I was going to be gone.

Interviewer: How did you know the patient was ready?

Expert Nurse: He made it very clear that he was ready. He was asking a lot of questions. He had had a regular ileostomy a couple of years ago and had finally been persuaded that a continent ileostomy was going to be the greatest thing for him. Earlier I thought he was feeling helpless about the operation he had just had. He looked as though he felt crummy. Physically, he was sort of stressed looking, nervous looking. Furthermore, he was treating the whole thing physically very gingerly. He didn't need to be that gentle with it. So by the time he started asking questions he was feeling better physically, feeling like there was some hope that he would learn how to deal with this.

Summary Statement   Although it was obvious to this nurse that the patient was ready, an outsider would note that she could make this judgment because she was so much in touch with his progress. The nurse did not attempt to teach this patient earlier and she did not force information on him before he communicated his interest in hearing it.

Assisting Patients to Integrate the Implications of Illness and Recovery into Their Lifestyles

In patient-care situations where temporary or permanent disability is all that can be hoped for, the nurse often helps patients to maximize their ability to continue with meaningful life activities.

EXEMPLAR I

An expert nurse described the role she played, early in her career, in helping a severely handicapped woman re-establish a meaningful life:

When I was very young, I worked for the Visiting Nurses Association. One woman I went to see on consultation hadn't been out of her bedroom for five years and was just dying of depression. She'd had a stroke and had not had much physical therapy. She had one completely frozen arm and very little mobility with her right leg. At the time, I knew very little about her chances for recovery. There were no orders for physical therapy. "Her heart is bad, the exercises might kill her," I was told. (Now you have to remember, that this was many years ago.) And I said, "She's dying anyway, she is dying because her whole world is just the four walls." And I wanted the opportunity to help, and I asked the doctor to give me the opportunity, by giving an order for physical therapy. And I promised to talk to the husband and to her about the fact that it is taking a big chance and that she may die. The doctor reluctantly gave me an order, and I exercised that woman, and got her out of bed. I got a book out of the library and read up on CVA physical therapy because I knew very little about physical therapy. She never regained the use of the hand and arm, of course, but she did get to the point that she could walk with help. And the first day she walked out of her bedroom, she just burst into tears. She died five and a half years later while cooking dinner. She had learned to peel potatoes with her one hand, wedging them against her paralyzed arm. She was a marvelous lady who was dying because she was being treated like an invalid, and she felt useless and hopeless.

EXEMPLAR II

Expert Nurse: This particular incident occurred when I was doing public health nursing. We would look through the cards we had in the clinic for all the health problems in the school. I found a card on a young man who was presently not in the classroom; he was being tutored at home because he was confined to a wheelchair. And he had a rare kind of progressive muscular dystrophy, and essentially what happened was that he was in the home because his father was unable to carry him into the station wagon and bring him into school. He had been confined to his home all summer. I went to the student director who was in charge of student welfare, and found out a little bit more about him, and found out that it was possible to go to the home. I did so, and found they had absolutely nothing in the home to assist him. His father carried him everywhere. They had some wheelchair ramps, but nothing in the bathroom, nothing outside. So I contacted the Muscular Dystrophy Association, and they came to the house, and they just did everything free — everything that was necessary. And they also provided transportation for him — whenever he wanted to go. He was very physically incapacitated — the disease was progressive and they had taken him to so many doctors, and he was quite debilitated because their current strategy, after trying everything else, was to have him on a whole bunch of vitamins and a vegetarian diet, so he was very, very deficient in a lot of things. Basically, my initial care consisted of getting his medical care up to snuff, which had not been done.

Interviewer: How did you do that?

Expert Nurse: Well, I talked to them [the family] a great deal. And what had happened was they had gone to so many different doctors who had told them that it was just hopeless. And so they were reading and they were sending away for different things, oh, you know, things like vitamin therapy, vegetarian diet, a holistic approach. They were looking for anything to give them some sort of hope. So the approach really was to try to improve his nutritional status. His hemoglobin really was very low. We just talked a great deal. Then he agreed to see some doctors. His diet was supplemented with vitamins and protein to make sure he was getting the proper amount of nutrients.

In talking with them, I found that his real love was radio announcing. He had a very nice voice. What he regretted more than anything about having tutors at home was missing his classmates at school. He was a senior in school and he loved being a spectator in sports, and had been, until the previous year, doing all the announcing at football games. And he had been unable to do this. I found a way to provide transportation to the games, and they set up the speaker system on a lower level that he could reach. And he continued after the first month to announce football games, and he was able to spend that year in school. He got much better medical attention, as well as filling his emotional needs of being with his peers.

Interviewer: If I'm hearing you right, now nobody was saying here's a problem that you should be interested in. What made you . . . ?

Expert Nurse: Well, I was looking at this card, and I guess the first thing was: "What is this condition documented here, and why can't he go to school?" And first approaching it from the fact of what is this disease, and what is being done for this child. To see if everything possible was being done. I found out that very little had been done, and felt it was very important to provide that—what was necessary and what this person needed. And I was quite surprised to find out that nothing had been done.

Interviewer: How long did your involvement with this family last?

Expert Nurse: To get everything implemented took two to three weeks. The Muscular Dystrophy Foundation was just phenomenal. And within about two months the home had been totally renovated. And within a couple of weeks' time he could go back to school and start announcing the football games.

> *Interviewer:*   What kind of difference do you think this made in this boy's life?

> *Expert Nurse:*   He smiled a lot more. He really blossomed. And he appeared to become stronger.

Summary Statement   In both exemplars, the nurses assessed the importance of trying to continue with normal activity versus the costs of inactivity and isolation. They also provided the patient and family members with alternative routes toward a more normal life despite the physical limitations.

Eliciting and Understanding the Patient's Interpretation of His or Her Illness

Nurses must remember, and expert nurses do, that patients often have their own interpretation and understanding of their condition. Allowing them to express this, as well as respecting and building on their interpretations, can play an important role in the patient's illness and recovery experience.

EXEMPLAR I

An expert clinician described how she elicited a young woman's interpretation of her breast cancer.

> *Expert Nurse:*   The patient told me a lot about her past sexual experience and how she didn't want to have a child but that she is very easily dominated. And so she had a child, not wanting to have it, and at this particular time she was feeling the reason for

her cancer was because she had a child. She felt this would not have happened had she not given in to her husband to have this child.

Interviewer: How did you respond to that?

Expert Nurse: I listened. I said, "It must be really hard for you to have a lot of guilt like that to carry around with you, if you think that this is the cause of your illness." And she does.

Interviewer: Was she asking you in any way if the pregnancy caused the cancer, or did you get the feeling that she was just sharing her thoughts with you?

Expert Nurse: Just sharing.

EXEMPLAR II

The patient was a woman in her mid-thirties with ulcerative colitis who had just had part one of a two-step operation. Part one involved creating a rectal pouch (similar to a continent ileostomy except that the person retains rectal control and has no stoma). The person has a temporary ileostomy for a few months, which is then reconnected to the lower bowel. This woman was at the point where she had an ileostomy that she would have to take care of for several months. She was willing to learn how to take care of it, but made no bones about the fact that she thought it was disgusting.

I taught her how to change her ileostomy bag and do skin care around the stoma. I didn't make any attempt to get her to feel differently about her ostomy. I respected her point of view that it disgusted her, but that she would learn to take care of it anyway. I made sure that she understood the anatomy and function, the simplest ways to care for it, and made suggestions to her that would make it less visible (e.g., covering it with a cloth bag, since she didn't like touching the stoma directly, she could remove the old bag and clean the skin around the stoma while she was in the shower). I think I made a difference by accepting where she was and teaching her with that in mind rather than trying to convince her that there was nothing wrong with the ileostomy and that she shouldn't be disgusted. (Interviewer note: This patient let the nurse know that her teaching had been particularly helpful.)

Summary Statement   The expert nurse in the first situation did not argue with the patient's interpretation of her illness. While acknowledging the difficulty and emotional pain that this interpretation must create, she just let the patient share this information with her, without quickly trying to convince her that this interpretation was wrong. This ability to elicit and understand a patient's interpretation is different from, although not unrelated to, the ability to *offer* an interpretation of a patient's illness, as discussed in the next section.

In the second exemplar, the nurse does not insist that the patient change her feelings about her ileostomy prior to learning how to take care of herself. She accepts the patient's interpretation and helps her work from that perspective.

Providing An Interpretation of the Patient's Condition and Giving a Rationale for Procedures

As there is increasing recognition of the fact that patients need and want to know what is being done to them and why, interpretation and explanation of procedures have become a key part of nursing activity. Discretion and skill are required. The nurse must assess how much information a patient wants and needs and find a vocabulary that the patient can understand. Sometimes, nurses must also acknowledge the limits of their own understanding.

EXEMPLAR I

It was a typical morning with doctors coming and going, patients going off to tests, etc., when I walked into one of my patients' rooms. A vascular surgeon and a neurosurgeon had just come out of her room. The patient was with her daughter and they were discussing the impending surgery. The patient was slowly going blind due to an aneurysm at the optic chiasma, and prior to coming to our hospital, the patient admitted her husband into an ICU in Santa Barbara with a heart attack. Under the circumstances, the patient was quite jittery—the surgery planned was a bypass of cranial arteries followed by a craniotomy to remove the aneurysm—after the pressure had been released around it.

I entered the room and asked how she was doing. Her first words were, "Should I have the surgery? Do you think it is safe?"

I replied, "You couldn't have finer surgeons than you have here and I can't make that decision for you."

She took a deep breath and began to express her many fears and concerns about the surgery. She expressed the thought that if she didn't have the surgery she would only get progressively more blind but still live. If she had the surgery she could die, she could go completely blind, she could be permanently disabled physically, or she could live with the remaining part of her vision. Instead of agreeing with her and interjecting my comments, I just kept silent. I felt that it was better to let her verbalize. After she had carried on this conversation with herself, I asked her if she would like me to explain what would be going on, to which she agreed. I took in Ichabod Crani—a plastic puzzle of the head with removable parts and identification of all the parts—brain, bone, veins, arteries, etc. In the next hour we played with the parts, and I answered her questions. By the end of the hour the patient had decided that since she had come all this way, she would go ahead with the surgery.

When I finally left the room, I felt that the patient had made the right decision but that she had made it on her own. I felt good because I had given her a very descriptive account, in terms she could understand, of what was to happen to her. I had tried to remain unbiased and open and answer her questions accordingly. It was a very positive experience and it seemed to be for her. Unfortunately, the surgery didn't go as well as we had all hoped. She eventually got better, with lots of care, and is now at a rehab hospital and recuperating remarkably well.

EXEMPLAR II

A Physician's Account of His Hospital Experience: All nurses coming on duty tried to make their own assessments of their patients' emotional level as well as their physical status. At times I would try to be falsely cheerful, and they would see through it. On one memorable Monday, I was obviously depressed, and my nurse, coming on duty, asked me gently what was wrong. I didn't have a clue. I wept buckets, something I don't usually do. I felt unashamed but puzzled. She said with some confidence: "We'll figure this out," and then went on to ask a few questions. She wanted to know, "Is the sound outside disturbing you?" I realized that it was. After a little further thought she said: "That is the wrecking ball knocking down the rest of old Bellevue. You didn't hear this noise Saturday and Sunday, but you did hear it Friday when your aortic balloon came out. That was a bad time. You remember not only how painful that was but you also remember how the balloon sounded inside you during all those rough days. I bet you are remembering all that pain." My distress disappeared. Another time when I seemed to be made uneasy by piano music played on my cassette player, a nurse pointed out that the same cassette had been played for me during one of my painful early weeks and that, again, it might be reminding me of those days. It was several more weeks before I was able to listen to any classical music without apprehension (Kempe, 1979).*

Summary Statement The nurses in these cases, aware that the patients were "tracking" their own progress or lack of it, responded fully and cogently to their requests for explanations.

The Coaching Function: Making Culturally Avoided Aspects of an Illness Approachable and Understandable

Illness, pain, disfigurement, death, and even birth are by and large culturally avoided and uncharted experiences. It makes little adaptive sense for the lay person to prepare in advance for the multiple, possible experiences of illness they may have, since illness and pain tend to be segregated, isolated experiences. Nurses, in contrast, through their education and experience, develop ways to observe and understand many ways of experiencing and coping with illness, suffering, pain, death, or birth and to offer patients avenues of understanding, increased control, acceptance and even triumph in the midst of these foreign, uncharted happenings.

Experience in addition to formal educational preparation is required for the development of this competency, since it is impossible to learn these ways of being

*Kempe, C. Henry, "A Personal View," *University of California, San Francisco Magazine*, Vol. 2, No. 2-3, June–September, 1979.

and coping with an illness solely by precept. A deep understanding of the situation is required, and often the ways of being and coping are transmitted without words but by demonstration, attitudes, and reactions.

EXEMPLAR I

A nurse clinician describes an encounter with a young man close to her own age who was visiting his dying father. The latter's condition suddenly deteriorated and the family was extremely distraught. The son stopped the nurse in the hall and asked how long his father would live. The nurse answered that she really didn't know, that it could be minutes, hours, days or weeks — there was no way to tell. He then asked if there were other dying patients on the unit. To which the nurse responded, "yes." She recounts the incident:

There was a long pause. Then he began a barrage of questions: "How could I work here; How can I go home and sleep at night; How could I do what I do?" No one had ever been so direct with such questions as these before, and their bluntness threw me off balance. But he was sincere and was *waiting* for my answer and so I told him how I had resolved these same questions within myself. It was not quite a monologue, but for 10 plus minutes he listened intently as I told him my feelings and my philosophy about life and about dying and about nursing. I told him how gradually I had settled into the medical floor instead of using it as a stepping stone to a surgical floor (which was my first intention). I told him how it *was* difficult, and how it *was* emotionally draining, and how it sometimes was difficult to sleep at night. I told him how there was gratification in helping a patient through the particular passage known as death and how I felt I was able to help the family also through the pain of that passage. I told him the gratification, the thing that kept me here, was in knowing that maybe somehow, I had made this particular rocky road a little smoother for those who had to travel it. With that, he hugged me, said "thank you" and turned away nodding his head, with tears in his eyes. There were tears in my eyes, too.

Summary Statement   In translating for the son how the culturally avoided had become understandable and approachable, the nurse broadened this young man's perspective and acceptance. This is what is meant by the coaching function of nursing—nurses who have come to grips with the culturally avoided or uncharted and can open ways of being and coping for the patient and the family.

In a second exemplar of this same area of skilled practice, a nurse offers us insight into a time of critical learning for her, a time when the patient gave *her* a new understanding of the ability to live and even enjoy life in the face of very extreme disfigurement, pain, and illness.

EXEMPLAR II

A young woman of 35 was admitted to the ICU. She had been diabetic since childhood, and because of that disease, she was now blind. She had had a right eye enucleation and a right leg amputation below the knee, as well as other surgery. As if that were not enough, she was admitted to the hospital for a heart attack. When the nurse first met this young woman, the patient was disoriented and had to be restrained. There was a feeling among the staff that the patient's physical deterioration was so extreme that maybe it would be better for her to

die. They felt it was a shame that technical intervention was keeping this woman alive.

The nurse described taking care of this young woman
during this phase and the change in her own attitude
when the patient regained consciousness and became
oriented again:

> Speaking with this woman I never saw such a feeling of wanting
> to live. Even with all that had gone on with her—all the
> destruction to her body—she had the most lovely personality that
> I had ever met. Her family also wanted us to do everything
> possible to keep her alive. The young woman said to me that she
> had a very hard time convincing people that she wanted to live.
> She told me of an experience at diabetic camp where they were
> afraid to let her come because they were afraid her diabetes
> would get out of control. The young woman told them, and this
> helps even in our unit, that if they came upon her and she was
> dead, they should remember that she died happy . . . She really
> impressed me. It was easy to take care of her after that. I brought
> books in, and we took turns reading to her with her family.

Summary Statement This is a powerful example because in it the nurse described an incident where her
own understanding expanded through being with someone with extreme handicaps. One can surmise that this
nurse drew on that experience thereafter. She had just
learned, in a very direct way, about a new kind of
possibility in the midst of deprivation.

We have collected many exemplars of this particular
kind of skilled nursing practice and are impressed that
in each case the nurse does not offer the patient precepts
or platitudes which might sound like: "Even in the
midst of great handicap and impossibility, I think it is
possible to make the most of it." That would be an

example of inflexible teaching by precept. But nurses, in the way they practice, by the *way* they approach a wound or the *way* they talk about recovery from a surgery, offer ways of understanding. And through the nurse's own ability to face and cope with the problem, such as a difficult, draining wound, the patient can come to sense that the problem is approachable and manageable.

In one small group interview session, the group agreed that one nurse's pre-op mastectomy teaching must be very effective, because her patient asked her if she herself had had a mastectomy. This nurse was very skilled and approachable in describing what the patient might expect after surgery, although the nurse had not had this surgery herself. She had learned from many patients a range of reactions and approximate time-tables for pain, recovery, and mobility after surgery.

| Summary and Conclusions

I am convinced that the five competencies listed in this domain represent only a fraction of the teaching-coaching competencies unique to the teaching–learning demands encountered by nurses working with the acutely ill. We have made progress in studying what information the patient finds most useful, but the results of such studies will always offer the more tangible, easily recognized learning needs. They will neglect the less tangible aspects of learning new ways to interpret bodily responses, new ways of being and coping with an illness. I think that nurses in labor and delivery have developed their role as "coaches" more fully than nurses in other specialities. We need to conduct descriptive ethnographies of effective and ineffective coaching strategies in the various specialties, both to refine and enhance these skills but also to recover and preserve this practical knowledge for our patients.

6 | The Diagnostic and Monitoring Function

The diagnostic and monitoring function of the nurse has expanded dramatically as the number of illnesses and interventions per patient have increased almost exponentially over the past 20 years. Many diagnostic tests and therapeutic interventions require careful monitoring, and the margins of safety are often narrow. The nurse taking care of transplant patients, for instance, soon learns to recognize early signs of infection and rejection. The nurse specializing in cardiovascular nursing learns to recognize the narrow zone between safety and toxicity for a number of potent cardiac drugs. And most specialties require close attention to fluid and electrolyte balance. The nurse's careful monitoring and early detection of problems are the patient's first line of defense. Many drugs can only be used safely if their effects are observed, if their possible incompatibilities, contraindications, and adverse reactions are caught early.

In fact, if the diagnostic and monitoring function of the nurse is not required, the patient is usually not hospitalized because the patient or his family can follow therapeutic instructions at home. Thus, diagnostic and patient monitoring functions are central to the nurse's role, yet even nurses fail to fully legitimize this role. In telling their stories of early warnings, nurses often told their stories as if they should not have been the ones to make the discovery. It was as if the nurses were saying, "In the best of all worlds, complications will not occur, and if they do, the doctor will be on the spot to pick up the first clues of patient deterioration." But, in actual practice, it is the nurse who spends the most time with the patient and who most often picks up the first clue. And that is as it should be.

We have much to learn from the wisdom embedded in the diagnostic and monitoring skills of expert nurses. Here the importance of perceptual abilities and of connoisseurship is central. Nurses with a background of experience with similar patients develop a specialized knowledge and a special language. By studying this language of the experts and by developing consensus about its usage, we will add to our clinical knowledge and point the way for others to gain the same perceptual skills (Benner & Wrubel, 1982).

For example, in a discussion of clinical knowledge development, nurses talked about learning to work in the "grey" zone where the patient changes were subtle and the margins of safety narrow. They recognized the importance of reacting quickly and appropriately without over-reacting. Unfortunately I was unable to pursue this "special language" of working the grey zone with its descriptive language of "aggressively chasing" (being ahead of the complications) or just "chasing" a problem (not keeping up with the patient's changes and not intelligently pursuing the problem), but I hope that other clinical researchers will be intrigued with the special language embedded in expert monitoring and diagnosis and with identifying more competencies (see box below) in this major domain of nursing practice.

Detection and Documentation of Significant Changes in a Patient's Condition

Nurses are most often the first to detect and document changes in a patient's condition. Unlike the early warning signal, to be discussed next, these changes can readily be documented by means of measurable vital signs and relatively clear observational data. This skilled performance includes clear documentation and presenting a firm, convincing case to the physician. The newly graduated nurse gaining expertise in this competency

Domain: The Diagnostic and Monitoring Function

Detection and Documentation of Significant Changes in a Patient's Condition

Providing an Early Warning Signal: Anticipating Breakdown and Deterioration Prior to Explicit Confirming Diagnostic Signs

Anticipating Problems: Future Think

Understanding the Particular Demands and Experiences of an Illness: Anticipating Patient Care Needs

Assessing the Patient's Potential for Wellness and for Responding to Various Treatment Strategies must master the recognitional component, the documentation, and finally the convincing presentation of the case. The first exemplar illustrates the mastery of this process.

EXEMPLAR I

Nurse:　When I first began, I found myself in a situation where the patient I was taking care of was behaving very strangely. Granted, it was a confounding situation. But I kept on running out of the room saying, "This is too weird." I really didn't make an assessment. In the beginning I would say, "Something is wrong in here," and go to somebody else, and they would say, "What are the patient's vital signs? What does the wound look like? What does the patient look like?" And I wouldn't have checked any of that. I would just say, "I think" or "I feel" that something's wrong. Whereas now I do a thorough assessment and contact the physician immediately, if warranted.

EXEMPLAR II

Expert Nurse:　I received a patient from CCU at about noon. She was an alert woman, in her 50s. I received a report from the CCU nurse stating that she was a post-MI, vital signs stable: pulse in the 80s, normal sinus rhythm, blood pressure between 120 and 130 (I don't recall the diastolic pressures). We made her comfortable in bed and checked her vital signs which were stable. About 30 minutes later, the patient had vague complaints of "not feeling well." Her blood pressure dropped to 110. Pulse was in the 90s, regular. I paged the intern and resident with no response. I finally reached the resident and reported my observations and told her the patient must be examined right away. She informed me she would be on her way to see the patient. I took another set of vital signs. The blood pressure had dropped to 104. Pulse remained the same. I noted that the patient was becoming "scared" by her facial expression. I had reassured her when she first complained that the doctor would be in to see her soon. During the whole episode, I asked an LVN to stay with the patient. I stopped the resident who was walking by and reported the drop in blood pressure and the patient's condition. She said she would be right back. I told her firmly to examine the patient now. She examined that patient and immediately paged another resident to check the patient. They stood outside the patient's room conferring on their findings. One said he heard a murmur; the other said she didn't hear it. While they were having their conference, I became very concerned about the patient's welfare. Time was slipping by since the onset of her complaints, and being a fresh post-MI, I felt she should be transferred back to CCU immediately. Since the onset of the patient's complaints to the time we transferred her back to CCU, it took 45 minutes. It was about 1:15 PM when we transferred her. At the end of my shift, I went to CCU to inquire about the patient. The nurses said they were still doing some tests to determine what was going on. Next morning I found out that the patient had died of a cardiac tamponade.

EXEMPLAR III

Participant Observation: Karen was doing a history and physical on a woman just admitted to the labor room. The woman's labor pains had ceased by the time she got into the labor room. After doing all of the history on the couple, she then checked the woman and found that true to the woman's history, she did have a retroverted uterus. She was dilated about one centimeter, and the cervix was ripe, soft. She compared what she found with what the doctor had found a week before. She said, "You have been doing something, but I don't think you're ready. You should go home and get some rest, because you will probably start labor within a day or so."

Summary Statement The patient assessment function of the nursing role has increased dramatically over the past 15 years. In these three exemplars the front-line assessment of the nurse is demonstrated to be central to optimal patient care. This competency not only has a recognitional component, but also requires expert documentation, and requires that the nurse present a convincing case to the physician.

Providing an Early Warning Signal: Anticipating Breakdown and Deterioration Prior to Explicit Confirming Diagnostic Signs

We have gathered a number of stories of the nurse anticipating deterioration before the evidence was convincing in terms of change in vital signs or other measurable evidence. When the stories are examined carefully, it is clear that the nurse is not using blind intuition, but rather is picking up on subtle changes in the patient's behavior or appearance.

EXEMPLAR I

Expert Nurse: We had a patient who had an esophageal dilatation in X-ray. She was a very uncomplaining woman of about 60 years of age. When she came back her vital signs were OK, and she was up in the bathroom. Later she started getting nauseated and she had streaks of very light pink drainage which I could account for by dilatation procedures, but I just had this feeling that something else was going on. She became worse; she became very nauseated. I called the house officer. Her vital signs were still stable, but I indicated that I wanted the house officer to check her. The house officer examined her but was not ordering any tests. I wanted to order blood work. I pointed out that the patient's nail beds were cyanotic. The house officer was unimpressed. It was almost time for me to go off duty when the patient started having chills with a temperature, so I called the house officer again and said there was something going on with this patient, and that I wanted to see something done for her before I went off duty. Later I found that the patient had a rupture in her esophagus; she also had aspiration pneumonia. Her pulse had gone up to 150. The house officer credited my persistence in getting early treatment in making a difference in the patient's outcome.

EXEMPLAR II

Expert Nurse: The LVN had one patient who was a pleasant elderly lady in isolation. She had had a cholecystectomy, been discharged, and had come back with a draining wound from the incision. This wound turned out to be a horrendous mess with fistulas and resistant bacteria. She had been on two or three strong antibiotics for some time and had diarrhea. I was in the room often because of her antibiotics, and she was becoming restless with a vague complaint of "not feeling good." Her color wasn't great and I started getting a "bad feeling" about this patient. I checked with the LVN on her midnight vital signs. She normally ran a low blood pressure (low 100s). We took the vital signs again and while they hadn't changed much, the systolic for the first time since admission was less than 100; it was 98. I then did a thorough assessment of her and found a small bruise in the groin that the LVN said had not been there before. That bruise shouldn't have been there. I called the doctor who was on call. He didn't know the patient, but I convinced him he really needed to see this patient even though it was 3 AM. By the time he arrived, all hell had broken loose. She was having copious burgundy liquid stools and the bruise in her groin had extended about a third of the way down her thigh. I started a second I.V. It was figured that her long course of antibiotics had killed her bacterial flora which had resulted in a Vitamin K deficiency and caused her bleeding. She ended up surviving after receiving, among other things, Vitamin K and blood products. But it was tight.

Summary Statement   There are a number of similar examples of early detection of a change in patient status before the presence of objective, measurable signs. This advanced recognitional ability frequently makes a critical difference in patient recovery. The effectiveness of this competency, however, gets linked with the nurse's skill in getting an appropriate and timely response from the physician.

Anticipating Problems: Future Think

One outstanding characteristic of expert nurses is that they spend a great deal of their nursing time thinking about the future course of a patient, anticipating what problems might arise and what they would do about them. Having seen many scenarios of patients, they are equipped with reality-based expectations and concerns for the ones they are currently dealing with. Their anticipation is very contextual, however. It is based on what they observe to be occurring with a *specific* patient, rather than what might happen to patients in general.

This competency includes giving forward-looking, problem-recognition reports to the oncoming shift of nurses. Some reports are retroactive descriptions of how the past shift went, which are seldom really predictive of how the next shift is going to be. But some nurses have the ability to present the report in terms of the situations most likely to develop and the problems awaiting resolution in the next 8 to 10 hours. For example, one nurse described her colleague's between-shift reports this way:

> If Sandra Smith is giving them report, then they do a better job that day, because she does the ground work for them. They don't have to go through the first hour of identifying problems. She has already done it. When she gives report, she tells them what she's handled and what still needs to be done. And she covers every aspect of every patient. It's phenomenal!

EXEMPLAR

Interviewer: When you are expecting a new patient in the ICU, what are you thinking about as you are getting ready?

Expert Nurse: Normally I'd be thinking about what their history is and what I might expect. Because the thing that saves me the most time, and the thing I try to teach people that I think helps them to get organized, and saves them the most time, is to think ahead about what might happen. Not necessarily *all* of the theoretical possibilities. But based on *this* patient. . . If I know something about the patient, I know what the pressure in their lungs is, what kind of surgery they're going to have, what their heart problem was, what their pulses felt like, whether their wife is worried or not, and I can pull all this information together and say: Probably this patient will bleed—they've had a high hematocrit and they might need some drugs to help cardiac output, so I'll mix those drips and have them ready, so if something happens I'm not trying to mix drips in the middle of it. So I get set for any eventualities that I think are likely to happen. Not something that *could* happen three percent of the time. But based on this patient's data, what I can expect.

Interviewer: So you're always living in the future?

Expert Nurse: Yes, and that's probably one of the big changes that's occurred in my practice over the years. Being able to make quick jumps on the basis of assessments that I don't have to think about anymore. I see it and can make it. And I'm able to project into the future. It's a very difficult thing to learn. It's hard sometimes for new nurses to put a group of facts together and come out with a process, to think about it. One can think in generalities, frequently: "Oh, I'm worried about urine output and kidney functioning," but it's much harder to take it a step further and ask, "How much intake am I going to give and how will I measure it? What criteria will I follow; what kinds of things will I see before that?"

Summary Statement   The expert nurse functions with an eye to the future. Many have learned the hard way that they must be ready for likely possibilities. Furthermore, expert nurses have multiple patient examples to call on that allow them to anticipate the course of a *particular* patient, based on that patient's *particular* history and current status. They are also able to translate current information into specific and detailed practical considerations they may have to face.

Understanding the Particular Demands and Experiences of an Illness: Anticipating Patient Care Needs

Expert nurses note that patients' long-term experience with a particular type of illness seems to create a particular approach to and definition of the illness by these patients. Several expert nurses noted that they could identify characteristic coping styles of patients with particular illnesses. They add that being aware of these identified styles enables them to understand the pa-

tients' interpretations of their illnesses and to anticipate their needs.

EXEMPLAR

Expert Nurse: We have a number of people coming in with
long histories of ulcerative colitis for surgery. They seem to be
much more compulsive in a lot of ways. They are people who
have been focused on their bodies for long enough that every
little change has more likelihood of being a big deal in the postoperative course than a lot of other people. Many of them are
young people who have been in the hospital a fair amount so that
they have a different picture of themselves vis-a-vis the hospital,
as opposed to other people who are in the hospital one time.
They are engulfed by their illness oftentimes, and in a sense more
dependent and demanding, but not in a way that would make
one real unsympathetic.

Interviewer: You said that you had some generalizations in
your mind about ulcerative colitis patients. How does that
translate into how you take care of them?

Expert Nurse: I give a lot more explanation about what's
happening with every little thing and why after surgery, trying
more to anticipate questions and fears. And I know I will need to
spend a lot of time teaching.

Summary Statement   Expert nurses seem to be able to
identify patterns of coping among patients with particular medical problems as well as to discern
idiosyncracies. Furthermore, they seem to be able to
translate these patterns into effective ways of working
with particular types of patients, ways that will minimize anxiety and maximize recovery.

Assessing the Patient's Potential for Wellness and for Responding to Various Treatment Strategies

Nurses in the psychiatric area, to be effective, must assess the patient's potential for wellness. This sense of what is possible for an individual serves as a guide for both treatment strategies and goals. The potential for wellness is not an ideal, but a realistic assessment based on a belief that an individual's life has possibilities even though it falls short of perfect wellness and adjustment.

EXEMPLAR

Expert Nurse: The doctor said, "We'll probably just keep her, discharge her tomorrow, I don't see any help for her." And I said, "I'm having trouble putting that together with the woman I saw this morning, because I saw her as somebody with potential and this is her first contact with psychiatry ever. She is really anxious to get some help. She is extremely bright even though her education is limited. And I see her as willing and anxious to grow and just needing desperately to have somebody to help her in this process." . . . I'm also quite confrontive and I really saw this woman as needing help, but the most important thing was, I saw her as somebody who was sensitive to what other people thought of her, and had so little ego, that if she went to that doctor and got the message, nonverbally or verbally, that she was helpless . . . And I told the doctor, "I think we have an obligation to give her the benefit of the doubt if nothing else, and if you really feel that she's hopeless, then my recommendation to you is that you get another doctor on the case, because she will pick up on your feelings. She is that sensitive, and she'll go with it and see herself as hopeless." . . . I said to him, "How long have you spent with her?" And he said, "Ten minutes." And I said, "Well, I think 10 minutes does not qualify you to decide if this is a hopeless case." . . . He talked with me afterwards; he said, "You know, I think you're right. I'm just amazed; she has really pulled herself together, and I see some strength and potential in her that I had not seen previously. I think we're going to keep her in the hospital for a few days and give her a chance to really do some work in the groups. I just wanted to tell you that I think you were right."

Summary Statement   In this exemplar, the nurse assesses the patient's potential for wellness and for responding to the proposed treatment strategies. All members of the therapeutic team have a responsibility to present their own perspectives and assessments of a patient and to document and report that assessment in an effective manner. In the psychiatric setting, it is not unusual for one team member to see a different side of the patient or have a different perspective than the others, based upon her or his particular relationship with the patient. Once nurses are convinced of their assessments, they are obligated to act as the patient's advocate in terms of that assessment or else reassess the situation.

Summary and Conclusions

In nursing process language, nurses' diagnostic and monitoring functions fit nicely into the assessment stage. However, this domain is so central and contains so much content and skill in its own right that much of the skill and content are overlooked if this domain is seen solely as the first step of a linear process.

We need to supplement the knowledge acquired through experience by systematically studying recognitional abilities and by increasing the accuracy and consensus of the descriptive language in this domain. The five competencies described in this chapter are only a beginning.

7 | Effective Management of Rapidly Changing Situations

Because it is the nurse who most often picks up the first signs of deterioration in a patient's condition, it is the nurse who must often manage rapidly changing situations until the physician arrives. One way to interpret this domain is simply to call it a "break in the system" and hope that future "breaks" can be avoided; this is an "incident report" approach. But such an approach produces a strange kind of fiction and an ineffective form of coping. It is fictional, for instance, to pretend that physicians will always be available when a patient's condition changes rapidly. Nurses *try* to detect changes early so that physicians will be available in the emergencies, and hospitals try to have backup physicians available at all times, but patient emergencies repeatedly outstrip the best of planning, and the nurse must manage until the physician arrives. Frequently this means that the nurse orders stat lab work or starts an intravenous line in anticipation of the need for emergency intravenous medications. This domain needs further documentation and legitimization so that nurses can be better prepared to perform in these emergency situations.

Hospitals have code blue teams available at all times, but many patient emergencies or "rapidly changing situations" fall outside resuscitation. A miscalled "code blue" can put the patient in new jeopardy. The exemplars in this domain (see list of competencies on page 111) illustrate that the nurse coordinates and marshals the support of other health team members. In a full-blown emergency, the nurse functions as the generalist, coordinating the functions of the various specialists. The patient is indeed fortunate if an experienced nurse is available to oversee the whole picture so that errors and duplication of efforts are prevented in situations where rapid responses are imperative.

Skilled Performance in Extreme Life-Threatening Emergencies: Rapid Grasp of a Problem

This area of skilled practice includes the ability to grasp the problem quickly, to intervene appropriately, and to assess and mobilize the help available.

EXEMPLAR I

Expert Nurse: At approximately 7:30 PM on a Friday afternoon, the Emergency Room was busy. Many of our staff were tied up in the major trauma room with an automobile accident. At this point the paramedics arrived with a 50-year-old woman who was complaining of chest pressure which had begun while she was gardening. Premature ventricular contractions were treated at the scene with a Lidocaine bolus, and an I.V. was running. I met the patient and the paramedics at the door and began talking to the patient. As we entered Room 2 the patient said, "I'm going to faint." The monitor showed ventricular fibrillation. I instructed the paramedic to begin chest compression as I rushed to plug in the defibrillator and called for the physician. The physician arrived just as I was ready to defibrillate her and offered to intubate her. I indicated that I thought that wouldn't be necessary and went ahead with the defibrillation, since I knew the time of onset and wanted to interrupt the arrhythmia as soon as possible. I then defibrillated the patient who responded immediately. She, in fact, requested to go home for a shower. Her monitor showed a regular sinus rhythm, and her vital signs were within normal limits. This incident was satisfying because the patient made a full recovery. It turns out that her problem was the life-threatening arrhythmia and not a myocardial infarction. She was able to go home in three days.

Domain: Effective Management of Rapidly Changing Situations

Skilled Performance in Extreme Life-Threatening Emergencies: Rapid Grasp of a Problem

Contingency Management: Rapid Matching of Demands and Resources in Emergency Situations

Identifying and Managing a Patient Crisis Until Physician Assistance Is Available

---

EXEMPLAR II

Expert Nurse: A 60-year-old female was received from paramedics in the Emergency Department with massive trauma

111

to pelvis and upper thighs as a result of a shotgun blast. Paramedics were infusing Ringers Lactate in the peripheral vein through a large bore catheter at a fast rate, and patient presented with good vital signs and appropriate sensorium. The Emergency Department doctor examined the patient briefly and requested orthopedic consult; he gave no initial order for treatment and promptly left the room. I suggested we start a second line, get a type and cross-match for several units of blood, and initiate the X-rays. The doctor agreed to the lab work and X-rays but felt we didn't need a second line or a CVP as the patient "looked good." I ordered the X-rays and lab that I felt were indicated and applied manual pressure as often as was possible to the open, oozing wounds of the pelvis and thighs. The patient became increasingly restless, anxious, thirsty, clammy, and vital signs fluctuated erratically depending on amount of fluid infusion. I informed both the Emergency Department doctor and the orthopedic doctor that I felt this patient was very hypovolemic and needed to go to surgery as soon as possible. Neither doctor seemed overly concerned and they reassured me the patient would do "fine." Initially the orthopedic doctor told me the patient would be going to a room upstairs before going to O.R. a few hours later. I lost my temper at that point and said that was ridiculous as this patient would not survive a few hours! The doctor then told me he'd see what he could do about moving up the operating room time and to just keep giving the patient fluids. At one time the patient's blood pressure dropped to 70 systolic and at that time I decided to start a second line and infused Ringer's Lactate as rapidly as I could with a corresponding rise in blood pressure. Approximately one hour after arriving in the Emergency Department, my patient was transported to the operating room. The patient arrested as they placed her on the operating room table, but fortunately was resuscitated. The surgeon apologized to me later and agreed that this patient was very hypovolemic and that he should not have procrastinated. I knew from the onset that my patient was literally exsanguinating in front of me and I felt totally frustrated in my attempts to get her doctors to see that. I did appreciate the surgeon's apology as that probably was a difficult thing for him to do. He also took the time to praise my nursing practice and stated that he thought I had kept the patient alive at least until she reached the O.R.

Summary Statement   In the first exemplar, the nurse grasps the importance of immediate intervention since she saw the transition into ventricular fibrillation. In the second exemplar the nurse grasps the importance of starting a second I.V. before the circulation is further compromised. This is an example of a competency available primarily to the expert.

Contingency Management: Rapid Matching of Demands and Resources in Emergency Situations

Nurses are most continually present on units and are most often aware of the total picture. Expert nurses often noted how they are aware of the rest of the staff, the total picture of patient needs, and the resources available to them. They are the overseers of the total picture; they are aware of and use the layers of available resources.

EXEMPLAR

An expert nurse described the following typical/atypical day in an emergency room.

Expert Nurse: This was a Sunday, 3–11 shift in the emergency department—going smoothly until approximately 9 PM—one medically urgent patient in the large treatment room; another chest pain arrives by private car and a severe asthmatic patient by the same mode; two ambulance rings down — another chest pain and a G.I. bleed. All four nurses are tied up assessing and initiating treatment; ambulance rings down — insulin shock coming in — goes to Trauma Room — two nurses needed — 17-month-old baby arrives by private car with febrile seizure — call the supervisor. Male arrives by private car — O.D. of pills and booze, very belligerent patient; is in large treatment room and must be moved to Trauma Room I. Move asthmatic and G.I. bleed to holding room with one nurse — G.I. bleed is to go to X-ray for arteriograms. Supervisor and one nurse are in Trauma Room with seizure and insulin shock — both patients are becoming stabilized. Medically urgent case has been seen by consultant, is ready for admission to ICU. Belligerent patient moved to private room. Consultant seeing most severe chest pain — to go to CCU. Febrile seizure to go home.

This type of two hours spent in an emergency room is typical. One must continually assess the state of the unit and keep the flow going. Nursing does this since the physician seldom knows the overall picture.

EXEMPLAR II

An expert nurse described her role in handling an emergency situation in ICU.

Expert Nurse: So we had most of the details taken care of by now. Someone is talking to the patient, someone's pumping blood in, another person has his finger in the dike (applying pressure to the point of bleeding), and another person is making sure that the patient is being ventilated.

Summary Statement   In these two examples we see how expert nurses function as orchestrators of a complex situation, keeping all fronts going, all bases covered. They are particularly able to single out the problems that need managing, to set priorities quickly, and to delegate responsibility for them to the available staff. They know how to function in the face of unpredictable situations and adjust their plans to the contingencies of the situation. Furthermore, they have confidence in their own ability and rarely panic in the face of a breakdown. It takes many straws to break the backs of experts.

EXEMPLAR III

Jolene, an expert nurse working in the ICU and actively struggling to save the life of a patient with a carotid bleed, did not panic when she heard there was no blood in the blood bank for the patient. Instead, she quickly mobilized the right person to take care of the situation, which helped both the patient and the panicked ICU resident.

Expert Nurse: By this time the problem is blood, we need blood, and so I said, "OK, someone call the blood bank and get us some blood." And the nurse said, "We just called and there's none down there." No one had caught that the patient was sitting up there with no blood in the blood bank. So we took off a blood (sample) from the arterial line and sent it down for a type and cross match. Meanwhile I started plasmanate and lactated Ringers, because the mean pressure was dropping down to about 30 and the blood was just pumping out of his mouth. About this time the ICU resident came in. He said, "What shall I do?" And I said, "You need to go down to the blood bank and get some type-specific blood for this patient, because a nurse can't get that. You're the only person who can get type-specific blood." It was the best thing he could do under the circumstances. I said, "Bring

115

two units, they will only give you two at a time, no matter how bad. But bring two and get back here as soon as you can." So he took off. (The patient's fluid resuscitation was successful and the bleeding was controlled enough to get the patient to surgery in time to repair the artery.)

Summary Statement   Their rich backlog of experience enables expert clinicians to create order in the midst of chaos. They have a variety of choices available to them and a sense of being at home in the situation.

Identifying and Managing a Patient Crisis Until Physician Assistance is Available

Nurses are often confronted with medical crises that require immediate medical attention; for example, it is most frequently a nurse who initiates a resuscitation effort. Considerable knowledge and skill are called for to determine the gravity of the situation and the necessity of rapid intervention—what can and should be started while waiting for a physician response. In these situations, the nurse walks a fine line between not jeopardizing the patient's life by withholding necessary life support measures and at the same time working within the bounds of safe nursing practice.

EXEMPLAR I

Expert Nurse: I came on duty at 3 PM and was assigned to a fresh postop open heart surgery. The patient had returned to the ICU around 11 AM that day and had all the usual paraphernalia for postops—I.V.s, respirator, chest tubes, foley catheters, etc. The patient had had a log of I.V. fluid and blood replacement on days—this is the usual procedure for open heart surgery—give lots of fluid at first (usually have had mannitol), then level off. Blood pressure will drop as the patient begins to warm up and dilate peripherally, but will usually level off soon. However, this patient continued to be hypovolemic—low blood pressure, low central venous pressure—and was diuresing in enormous amounts. We were pouring fluids in, in an attempt to catch up, but were managing, barely, to stay even with output. The patient by this time (4:30–5 PM) was fully warm, so clearly something else was amiss here. I telephoned the surgeon's exchange but was not able to locate him. The exchange promised that they would have him call as soon as possible. I tried also to contact the assistant, but he was off call to another doctor who was not terribly familiar with open heart surgery. Meanwhile, we were pouring in fluids, blood and packed cells, without orders, just to stay even, for the patient was continuing this diuresis. I began reviewing the possible causes for this and decided a likely one was hyperglycemia. I then ordered a blood glucose level and the results came back—more than 600 mg percent. About this time the assistant surgeon had come back on call and I was finally able to contact him. He prescribed for the patient on the basis of the blood glucose level and we were then able to stabilize the patient.

Summary Statement   This nurse recognized the relative period of time in which intake and output equilibrium should have been established. She was able to consider a somewhat unusual cause for this — one that a less experienced nurse could not be expected to consider. She was confident enough to act without doctor's orders; on her own, she ordered fluids, blood, and lab tests. She saved approximately one hour in diagnosis of the patient by having the glucose test results when the physician was available.

EXEMPLAR II

Expert Nurse: We go into the delivery room . . . two of them were already being used so we had our C-section room that we reserve for C-sections that was not at all set up—had no instruments. We wheeled the bed into the room and the lady is pushing and stooling at the same time on me, and here comes the head. And I said, "Doctor, don't take time to wash your hands." . . . I told the nurse's aide that she had to come with me first, and she gave me a pair of gloves and a set of instruments and this baby came flying out in my hands, and meanwhile the doctor is washing his hands. And so I sucked the baby up, and thank God, it was a big baby or I don't know what I would have done had it been two months early as had been predicted. We got the baby's cord clamped. She was fine; she was wonderful.

EXEMPLAR III

Expert Nurse: I had just admitted a new patient with the diagnosis of GI bleed. The doctor had given minimal orders as "he would be right over." Well, the doctor's "right over" turned into a fair amount of time. The patient's blood pressure was in the 100s and his pulse in the 90s and he seemed fairly stable. He turned on his call light and stated he felt a little nauseated. He promptly had a huge emesis of dark brown burgundy. What skin color he had drained almost instantaneously away and the sweat popped out in beads in its place. I laid him back down, told one nurse to get a blood pressure, and another to start an I.V. of normal saline. I called the doctor but the exchange said he was "off call." The on-call doctor was angry, saying he hadn't been told he was covering for this doctor, that he didn't know the patient, and refused to give orders. I told the exchange to put me through to the primary physician. They said he was in transit. I then ordered a packed cell volume and hemoglobin, three units packed cells, and lab work to see if there was a coagulate deficiency. I then started a second I.V. and iced saline washes

118

through a nasogastric tube. The doctor finally did show up. I told him what had been done and this was fine with him. I then asked him to be sure to sign off the orders.

Summary Statement These three exemplars illustrate that the nurse must possess a high degree of expertise to identify a patient crisis accurately and manage it effectively until a physician is available. This area of nursing functioning is fraught with ambiguity, but the prevalence of such patient care situations and the importance of this nursing competency to the patient's welfare call for increased legitimization and clarification of this function.

Summary and Conclusions

Nurses must be able to manage as well as prevent crises. We create fictions for our discipline if we hold an idealized view of preventing crises that blocks systematic description of the nurse's performance in actual crises. We cannot afford to relegate a major area of our actual performance to "non-nursing" or "incident report only" status. Since the nurse is the one who is present at the patient's bedside and since one of her major functions is to diagnose and monitor patient changes, it follows naturally that the nurse will be required to manage rapidly changing patient situations. We contribute to the recognition lag in nursing when we fail to document and legitimize this major area of our actual practice.

8 | Administering and Monitoring Therapeutic Interventions and Regimens

Procedural descriptions of the competencies in this domain (see box on page 123) can be found in almost any procedure book, but the exemplars in this chapter illustrate the additional demands, resources, and constraints that come into play when the particular patient and particular context are taken into consideration. Nurses often fail to give themselves credit for their skill in administering the often complex and intricate current therapeutic interventions and regimens. Many of these interventions have been delegated to the nurse in an ad hoc fashion; and in their wake, new practices and skills are developed — also passed on in ad hoc ways. We have had numerous "time-motion" studies in nursing to assist us with cost containment, but we have had almost no systematic description of the skilled practices that have evolved as a result of new therapies. Newly graduated nurses find that actually doing the "procedures" they have been taught requires more varied and complex skills than they have learned in the nursing lab or through practice on one or two patients.

The administration of medication has become simplified by increased assistance from pharmacists. I can remember when hyperalimentation fluids were prepared on the units and required more precision, skill, and time than it takes to make a good German chocolate cake. Now a unit dosage system and pharmacist participation make drug administration safer and less time-consuming. However, the number of medications administered intravenously has increased, and these require close monitoring and sophisticated knowledge about possible incompatibilities and untoward effects. Nurses could significantly contribute to the knowledge of therapeutic and untoward responses to medication by systematically keeping a record of what they learn from their own practice.

The exemplars in this chapter *underrepresent* the large amount of knowledge embedded in this domain. They point the way toward treating our craft with greater respect by taking seriously our skills in administering and monitoring therapeutic interventions and regimens.

Starting and Maintaining Intravenous Therapy with Minimal Risks and Complications

Most patients receive intravenous therapy or blood products at one time or another during their hospital stay. Nurses become astute in tailoring I.V. placement, mode, and maintenance strategies based upon a number of variables such as patient mobility needs, condition of the veins, possible length of therapy, and the latter's nature and purpose. The applied technology of intravenous therapy has grown considerably. It is no small accomplishment today to learn how to pace I.V.

Domain: Administering and Monitoring Therapeutic Interventions and Regimens

Starting and Maintaining Intravenous Therapy with Minimal Risks and Complications

Administering Medications Accurately and Safely: Monitoring Untoward Effects, Reactions, Therapeutic Responses, Toxicity, and Incompatibilities

Combating the Hazards of Immobility: Preventing and Intervening with Skin Breakdown, Ambulating and Exercising Patients to Maximize Mobility and Rehabilitation, Preventing Respiratory Complications

Creating a Wound Management Strategy that Fosters Healing, Comfort, and Appropriate Drainage

therapy accurately, to administer a variety of medications and fluid products that may or may not be compatible, and to assess when an I.V. should be discontinued due to infiltration or phlebitis. In the first exemplar, the competency of starting and maintaining intravenous therapy with minimal risks and complications is made visible by a new nurse discussing her acquisition of this knowledge.

EXEMPLAR I

New Graduate Nurse: There are a lot of tricks of the trade when it comes to I.V.s. When I was team leading on days, we were responsible for all the I.V.s and all the meds on one side and I would go to my preceptor and say, "Why won't this I.V. go?" And she would come in and raise the I.V. up a little and play with the tubing—things that I didn't know how to do—and I would turn around and find that it was going. Otherwise, I would just be wondering, "Why won't it go?" She really knew the tricks and that helped a lot. That was very helpful, because a lot of times it just won't go, and sometimes it's just positional, things like that. And I would say to her, "There's something wrong with this I.V., and she would say, "Have you tried this and have you tried that? Have you raised the bottle? Have you repositioned the arm? Have you done this?" She was really helpful about that.

EXEMPLAR II

A preceptor talks about passing her clinical knowledge on to a beginner:

Interviewer: What are the kinds of supervisory help that the new graduate needs with I.V. therapy?

Preceptor: They have a lot of questions. How do you choose between a butterfly or an I.V. intracath? They have to consider why you want that line in. And just learning the insertion alone is difficult. You take into consideration the length of time you will be leaving the line in and the kinds of medications that will be given, or whether it's a short-term, keep-open I.V. With limited medications, then the butterfly I.V. is more comfortable and presents less of a threat of phlebitis. Doctors vary in their preferences as well, and you have to take that into consideration. And of course, the condition of the patient and his veins makes a great deal of difference. For example, with older patients special skill is required. They look as if they are going to be so easy to get in because the veins look large, but they are so fragile. If you do not use a very, very slight tourniquet, the thin membrane of the older patient's vein will just pop open.

Summary Statement   These two exemplars demonstrate the nuances involved in mastering the technology of intravenous therapy. Once this competency is mastered, it is difficult for the proficient nurse to recapture the stages of learning the skill.

Administering Medications Accurately and Safely: Monitoring Untoward Effects, Reactions, Therapeutic Responses, Toxicity, and Incompatibilities

The nursing responsibility for monitoring the safety and therapeutic responses to medication has grown with the development of more potent drugs and the proliferation of new medications with limited clinical track records. Indeed, the rationale for hospitalization may frequently be to have expert nursing observation and documentation of responses to medications, so that therapeutic levels can be determined. While sophisticated laboratory tests usually provide the final documentation, it is the nurse who discovers the need for the laboratory tests. Here, expert clinical assessment over time is crucial to patient safety and even recovery.

EXEMPLAR I

A psychiatric nurse is being observed while administering medication.

A young male patient came up to receive his medication, and she asked him how the tremors were in his jaw. He gave an elaborate description of how the roof of his mouth quivered and was connected to his brain. The nurse later explained that she had just noticed the quivering of his jaw a couple of days ago and was concerned that he had tardive dyskinesia — irreversible damage caused by psychotropic drugs. The doctors had taken him off his psychotropic medications and had started Cogentin to see if the symptoms would recede. She said that it is very hard to discern what is going on because the patient incorporated the symptoms of the medication reaction into his delusional system.

EXEMPLAR II

Expert Nurse: I was in charge on evenings and was making rounds. On the prior night shift they unfortunately had a float charge nurse, and she had hung a Lidocain I.V. drip using a macro-drip chamber instead of a micro-drip chamber. During that shift the patient was not responsive, but he had been a little confused before, so they didn't really make too much note of it. He was on the monitor but there were no changes there. During the day shift a new graduate nurse was working with him because the head nurse and the assistant nurse were not there. And she didn't even notice the macro-drip chamber. So I made rounds, noting that in report they had said the patient was even less responsive. On rounds the first thing I saw was that there was a macro-drip chamber and Lidocaine was being administered. I am alert to this error because once I almost made the same error. Unfortunately, this incident did not have a happy ending. I turned off the medication, but the patient had started having widened QRS waves, and then had a cardiac arrest. We were not able to resuscitate him.

EXEMPLAR III

Expert Nurse: I had taken care of Mrs. X, a 64-year-old postop patient, for 7 of her 10 days of hospitalization. One morning after I had helped her to walk a bit and settled her into her chair and was making her bed, we were chatting as usual – we liked each other. I noticed she was mistaking things that I would say for something else. Mrs. X was on day 10 of a 14-day course of streptomycin. I knew, of course, that streptomycin could cause eighth cranial nerve damage, but I had never seen a patient in which this had occurred. But I was sure Mrs. X couldn't hear me as well as she could last week. After talking this over with the charge nurse, I called the doctor and told him my observation. He was skeptical, but agreed to see the patient before the next dose of streptomycin. Early this afternoon, Mrs. X's daughter visited. I noticed her going down the hall, so I called her aside and asked her to see if she thought her mother's hearing was different from before. Realization that there was a problem flooded the daughter's face. She had noticed the problem, but had not been conscious of it until I mentioned it. Anyway, to make a long story short, the doctor agreed that Mrs. X had suffered some hearing loss, and decided that he was able to discontinue the streptomycin so that no further damage was done.

Summary Statement　These three exemplars illustrate a range of observations and significant implications for accurate and safe administration of medications. This competency includes not only the accurate and safe administraton of medications, taking into consideration possible drug interactions or incompatibilities, but also requires that the nurse expertly monitor untoward effects, reactions, therapeutic responses, toxicity, and incompatibilities. Such monitoring, as these exemplars show, can have life and death implications.

Combating the Hazards of Immobility

Many nursing interventions are related to preventing the hazards of immobility created by the patient's illness or by therapeutic interventions. The skilled nursing involved is varied and takes into consideration the maintenance of a healthy intact skin, maximum range of movement, paced ambulation, and respiratory therapy to maximize ventilation and pulmonary hygiene. But in each case the nurse must assess what is needed, as well as motivate the patient and provide appropriate pain management strategies.

EXEMPLAR I

Participant Observation: Ellen was providing information on a patient to a physician. There was a friendly exchange, collaborative I think, between this physician and nurse. Ellen showed the doctor the new kind of plastic strip wound healing material that she had put on the patient's buttocks for the decubitus that had developed there. Ellen explained that she had gone to an ostomy conference on it. It had been used in England for a number of years, she said, and it had just been introduced here. She explained that it attracts serum to the area, and went on to explain the theory behind the dressing's purported effectiveness. This intervention was added to a number of strategies that the nurses were using to prevent skin breakdowns on this patient (e.g., frequent turning, massage, air mattress).

EXEMPLAR II

Participant Observation: Elizabeth approached the bed of Christine, a very frail, middle-aged woman. She asked, "Do you want to walk now?" Christine nodded her head vehemently no, but with a smile in her eyes. Elizabeth responded, "When am I going to learn to tell you and not ask you!" Elizabeth came back with what seemed to be an appropriate order, "It is time for you to walk." With a bit of delay, insistence, and humor from Elizabeth, Christine was soon up and walking, though liking it very little.

EXEMPLAR III

Participant Observation: Nora approached the patient's bedside and said, "I haven't seen you do your breathing exercises today." The patient indicated that it hurt too much to use the ball spirometer and that he wasn't up to it. Nora asked if he was having much pain. When he said that he was, she offered to give him some pain medication, and indicated that he could try doing the coughing and deep breathing as soon as he was more comfortable. She emphasized that it was very important that he exercise his lungs.

Summary Statement   These exemplars illustrate a range of nursing interventions to prevent the hazards of immobility. As illustrated, *strategies* for managing pain and supporting patients through uncomfortable activity are required. Successful motivation and timing of these nursing interventions are crucial.

Creating a Wound-Management Strategy that Fosters Healing, Comfort, and Appropriate Drainage

In many areas of nursing, nurses care for patients' wounds; available to them is an array of dressing materials and ointments. These are used often routinely and many times creatively, to assure a clean wound that heals quickly. In this area of skilled performance, assessment of the different kinds of drainage and their treatment implications is critical. This area of skilled performance is illustrated in the following two exemplars:

EXEMPLAR I

Participant Observation: Diane returned to the bedside of a
new patient after a group of physicians had finished their
procedures for the patient. They had removed all of the patient's
dressing exposing a belly with six abdominal wounds. Diane
spent the first hours of her shift trying to clean up the area and bag
those wounds. This first entailed removing aluminum paste
which had been applied in some places as a skin protector. Some
of the wounds had irrigating catheters in them, some of them did
not. There were bilateral abscesses and one of them was putting
out big clots of blood. The nurse talked to the patient all through
the procedure, reassuring him. Even though the patient was only
semi-conscious, he later stated that he remembered her voice and
her reassurance. She assessed the type of drainage and the
effective bagging and tube placement for each type of drainage.
Skin protection strategies were also varied depending on the
nature and location of the drainage. Upon completion she wrote
up a description and wound management plan for this patient,
who after several months improved enough to be able to
go home.

EXEMPLAR II

Expert Nurse: I was taking care of a 40-year-old female who
had been hospitalized for 3 months in another hospital and came
to our hospital the day before to have her abdominal fistulas
corrected. The night before I met her, the bag collecting her
fistula drainage fell off three times and was reapplied the same
way each time by her nurse due to the patient's insistence that
nothing else works. Her skin was very excoriated in spots and
was very tender. She was upset that nothing was working and
was afraid to move because of the drainage increasing with
activity. I removed the leaking bag and saw that the problem was
that she had a large crease between two recessed fistulas. She
was resistant to my suggestions, so I told her that she should trust

me because I've had numerous similar situations that I've had positive outcomes with. She said, "You mean you've seen a mess like this before? This bad?," and I told her that that was our specialty here and that I was sure I could get a bag to stay on her for at least 24 hours, if not more. She said she'd love it to happen and said I could do what I wanted. She questioned all of my actions and was a bit resistant to a few suggestions and changes that I made, but I was persistent and acted very confidently about my success with such cases. I would use stomahesive paste to fill in her crevices and she'd say: "It never worked before." Then she'd say I was using too much, and I'd say that's probably why it never worked before—they never used enough. She was questioning a lot and as a result she learned a lot about the application of the appliance—specific to her. I encouraged her participation. The bag remained on for 3 days and was removed to check out the skin underneath. When we reapplied the appliance, she participated in cutting out her pattern, suctioning the drainage while we aired her skin. She actually did a lot. Her skin improved and she felt better about the situation.

I think that my confidence and insistence were the key in her acceptance of my technique. I never really doubted that I could make it work and I feel I communicated it to her and felt that giving her all of the information that I had about the procedure, step by step, that her attention was redirected postively and constructively and made her more receptive. By my taking the role of teacher she became the "student" so to speak, and that gave me the control I needed and eliminated a power struggle with her. She also became a participant in her care and had some control over her situation with her information.

Summary Statement   In both these exemplars, the nurse's attitude and approach to dressing the patient's wound conveyed to the patient that the wound *was* manageable. A considerable range of products and materials is available to use in wound management, and the nurse's competency includes keeping up with the technology available. However, the effectiveness of the technical innovations depends upon nurses' knowing not only the latest research but also the art and skills of applying the technology.

Summary and Conclusions

The knowledge embedded in this domain is hidden by strictly procedural descriptions that do not take into account the variability and thoughtful adaptations that must be made in administering and monitoring therapeutic interventions. The craft and wisdom gained with experience in this domain are not adequately captured by interview or self-report, because nurses gain their skill through trial and error and are typically not aware of many aspects of this skilled practice. However, participant observation of many nurses at different skill levels can uncover some of the intricacies and variability in actual practice.

Often therapies are designed with little consideration of the actual implementation or delivery of the therapy. The latter is left for the nurses to design in the field. Once the innovations surrounding the implementation are in place, they are taken for granted with few avenues for describing the practical development involved.

Polanyi (1958) has pointed out scientists' inability to capture in formal terms much of what occurs in applied industrial settings. Therefore, I am not calling for more detailed procedural descriptions. Descriptive and interpretive accounts of the practical development and the variability in the skilled practices associated with administration and monitoring therapies would be useful. The variations, once adequately described, could then be compared in terms of effectiveness. The context would have to be taken into consideration since the therapies are administered to self-interpreting human beings who respond differently to ministrations that are delivered with care and concern in contrast to those delivered with indifference or carelessness.

9 | Monitoring and Ensuring the Quality of Health Care Practices

Because nurses are ever present and coordinate the multiple interactions the patient has with the health care team, they are in a position to prevent and detect errors; they are especially alert during the initial learning stages of new residents. In the interview sessions nurses talked about how much of their time was spent in preventing and spotting errors. They did not talk with pride about this skill. Instead, these competencies (see box on page 137) were not presented as competencies but as "system failures," akin to the emergency interventions described in Chapter 7. It was as if the system *should* be better and that potentially dangerous errors should never happen.

The nurses were visibly uncomfortable talking about this aspect of their role that takes a considerable amount of their time. The eminent physician and medical essayist Lewis Thomas (1983) describes this domain with ease and confers upon it the respectability that the nurses seemed reluctant to acknowledge. His observations come from the perspective of a physician and a patient:

My discovery, as a patient first on the medical service and later in surgery, is that the institution is held together, *glued* together, enabled to function as an organism, by the nurses and by nobody else.

The nurses, the good ones anyway (and all the ones on my floor were good), make it their business to know everything that is going on. They spot errors before errors can be launched. They know everything written on the chart. Most important of all, they know their patients as unique human beings, and they soon get to know the close relatives and friends. Because of this knowledge, they are quick to sense apprehensions and act on them. The average sick person in a large hospital feels at risk of getting lost, with no identity left beyond a name and a string of numbers on a plastic wristband, in danger always of being whisked off on a litter to the wrong place to have the wrong procedure done, or worse still, *not* being whisked off at the right time. The attending physician or the house officer, on rounds and usually in a hurry, can murmur a few reassuring words on his way out the door, but it takes confident, competent, and cheerful nurses, there all day long and in and out of the room on one chore or another through the night, to bolster one's confidence that the situation is indeed manageable and not about to get out of hand.

Knowing what I know, I am all for the nurses. If they are to continue their professional feud with the doctors, if they want their professional status enhanced and their pay increased, if they infuriate the doctors by their claims to be equal professionals, if they ask for the moon, I am on their side. (p. 679)

Thomas is correct to associate knowing the patient as a person with the prevention of errors. Commitment to the patient as an individual and engagement in the situation are required to produce sufficient cue sensitivity to detect potential errors (Wrubel, Benner, & Lazarus, 1981). The uninterested, disengaged nurse will not be alert to the unusual clues that signal trouble for the patient. Nurses also need a keen sense of the patient's usual behavior and appearance to detect subtle but significant changes.

Domain: Monitoring and Ensuring the Quality of Health Care Practices

Providing a Backup System to Ensure Safe Medical and Nursing Care

Assessing What Can Be Safely Omitted from or Added to Medical Orders

Getting Appropriate and Timely Responses from Physicians

Providing a Backup System to Ensure Safe Medical and Nursing Care

Sometimes the nurse is requested to set up an intervention on a patient that conflicts with safety standards or, in other situations, the previously adequate and safe plan of care must be changed as the patient's condition changes. It is the nurse who must therefore call for changes in the plan of care.

EXEMPLAR I

Expert Nurse: Frequently what happens in our work is that we're dealing with inexperienced physicians who know less than we do about what respirator changes to make on the premature infants. So what I feel is part of my job in critical care is to protect patients from physicians who are less experienced than I am on respiratory care. So I will anticipate that the physican is going to make such and such change based on this blood gas report. If he does *not* make such and such change, I'm going to ask him why. And if he can explain to me something that's logical and based on sound data, then I'll go ahead and do what he wants to do and have no qualms about it. If he's saying I *don't* know why, I'm going to insist that he go on to the next higher person on the line and find out. Or *I will!*

EXEMPLAR II

Expert Nurse: We had a patient come into the emergency room who looked very ill. His private physician was called. When I listened to his lungs, I could only hear air entry on one side. When the physician arrived, he decided that the patient was hyperventilating and requested a brown bag to have the patient breathe into in order to treat the "hyperventilation." The patient was obviously on his way to his death bed. I refused to give the brown bag and called the ICU and said, "You're going to get a patient. The patient is very ill. As soon as he arrives, I want you to call in the emergency panel physician." I did this because we were not getting through to this physician that the patient needed some morphine and some blood gases drawn. We had to decide whether we would try to alleviate his pain or try to make him better. It turned out that the patient died; his illness was irreversible. But at least the appropriate assessment and pain relief interventions were done.

EXEMPLAR III

Expert Nurse: I was specialing a patient this morning who had an arteriovenous shunt put in yesterday and her pressure was really low. By noon we transferred her to CCU for a dopamine drip, but initially we were having a hard time finding a bed for the patient. The physician wanted to start the dopamine drip on the unit where we had no cardiac monitoring capability. I knew it was risky. If we would have been unable to get a bed in CCU, I would have to get a portable cardiac monitor before initiating the dopamine drip.

Interviewer: Was it your sense in this situation that the physician was just expecting you to provide a monitor for the patient on the unit?

Expert Nurse: I think that their outlook is so medically oriented that the goal was to give the dopamine. They were not thinking of what it would be like to cart the patient down the hall four blocks if we got into trouble, or where we could get a monitor.

Summary Statement Nurses are often caught in the ambiguous role of serving as a back-up system to ensure safe medical and nursing care; often this entails altering the treatment plans of other care providers. Expert nurses are aware of the possible avenues for circumventing problems as they arise; they work with a healthy skepticism and ongoing questioning of treatment plans; and they are well aware of their capability to provide back-up safety and to change treatment plans as the patient's condition dictates. They know from experience that anyone can make mistakes, and they are able and prepared to act on their own judgments if necessary.

Assessing What Can Be Safely Omitted from or Added to Medical Orders

While medical orders provide the guidelines for many of the nurse's activities, nurses *must* use discretion in carrying them out. They are expected to assess what

139

they *should* do to provide the best possible care for the patient rather than simply carry out by rote medical orders, even though this may involve risks for them. This skill, at its simplest level, means that the nurse will discontinue orders which are clearly no longer relevant to the patient's well-being. But at its most complex level, as the exemplars illustrate, the skill involves a weighing of conflicting needs and deciding whether, for example, rest and emotional comfort are more healing at a particular time than the therapeutic regimen ordered.

This issue comes up frequently in intensive care units, where the problems associated with sleep deprivation may outweigh the problems incurred by withholding or delaying a treatment. Several nurses noted that with experience they tend to use more discretion in carrying out orders such as taking vital signs. In that case they talked about the value of assessing the need for the vital signs against the patient's need for sleep and rest. In all cases discretionary judgment was based on the nurse's understanding of many aspects of the patient's condition.

EXEMPLAR I

Expert Nurse: I took care of a patient, a very likable young physician, who had an open-and-close exploratory laparotomy for pancreatic cancer. He had been febrile. For three nights I woke him every four hours and helped him do all his breathing exercises and lung physical therapy. He was really depressed and wasn't talking about anything that had to do with his diagnosis and everything that was happening to him. The fourth night that I was on, his temperature had come down some, and by now he was exhausted from lack of sleep. I figured that he was going to have a lot better chance to focus on things that he needed and wanted to focus on if he could just get some uninterrupted sleep. His temperature remained the same in the morning. His lungs probably would have been clearer had I awakened him at 3 AM, but I elected not to, given his extreme fatigue and depression. It's not clear what is the right thing to do. There are little studies done about the effectiveness of chest physical therapy and then there are other studies done about the effectiveness of sleep. But there is never anything that proves that X is better than Y, especially in a particular situation, so that I know that chest physical therapy every four hours is really going to help or that sleep is going to help. It is expected that I will use my best judgment under the circumstances.

EXEMPLAR II

Expert Nurse: In the beginning, I was writing down all the times that blood pressures were to be taken, and then I thought, "Hey, wait a minute, let me think about this and decide whether I need to take them or not. After all it's not just something I'm supposed to do to make *me* feel better." So I stop and think, what if I know what someone's blood pressure is? What does that tell me? Do I really need to know it? Especially with some of the postoperative eye patients who have been postop for a couple of days. We are expected to use our judgment as to when to discontinue the vital signs at night. So we carefully study the trends and the patient. Sometimes I substitute close observations, so the patient can sleep.

Summary Statement   In both these exemplars, the nurse makes a judgment about the relative merits of rest and comfort over the prescribed therapy at a *particular* time in the patient's illness. There can never be precise scientific guidelines for these decisions, because there could never be enough research done to capture the particulars of all situations. The nurse will always need to be able to weigh the important against the important and, given the particular situation, risk choosing in the interest of the patient's well-being.

Getting Appropriate and Timely Responses from Physicians

If nurses are to get timely and appropriate responses from physicians, then they must communicate clearly and convincingly. They also need to know which alternative physicians should be called if the primary physician is unavailable. (Some hospitals have better support systems and backups than others.) Nurses talk about the art and skill of presenting a convincing case to a physician. They also talk about the value of knowing when to be adamant, of knowing the physician and his idiosyncracies, and of establishing their own credibility through their competence.

At times a physician will read a patient situation differently than the nurse and elect not to respond as requested. In these instances the nurse has to decide whether to use the appropriate backup medical consultation services available in the hospital to provide maximum coverage for the patient.

EXEMPLAR

Expert Nurse: A patient was admitted with a diagnosis of thrombophlebitis. He had been on heparin therapy for about two days when I first saw him. The report from the night shift said that he had had a difficult night. He had been having pain, more than usual. The intern on call was phoned, but did not come up to see the man. Instead Demerol was ordered I.M. Because the I.M. medication did not relieve the pain, the nurse phoned the intern again. By this time the nurse told the doctor that the patient was slightly short of breath. But the intern thought the nurse was being an alarmist and did not come up to see the man. The doctor then ordered Percodan. By 7 AM when I went in to see the patient, the man was clammy, cool, restless, and his vital signs were changing. He was more short of breath than had been described, was diaphoretic, had thready pulse, and was still in pain. I phoned the intern who regularly followed him and recounted the events of the night. He listened, paused, and then asked if I was calling to get more pain medication for the man. In a controlled manner I told him that something was going wrong with his patient and that giving him more narcotics would not solve the problem. I also said that I was calling because I wanted a doctor to see this man *NOW*. The intern came right up, and not a minute too soon. The man's level of consciousness was dramatically changing for the worse as were his vital signs. The intern phoned his resident. The patient had an infarction in his lung. Fortunately swift action was taken and a specialist was called who, through surgery, was able to save the man's life and lung. The intern thanked me for my persistence in getting the patient seen promptly.

Summary Statement   The problems inherent in getting an appropriate and timely response from a physician make this competency visible. Patient-care situations were frequently described where getting such a response was a key issue.

Summary and Conclusions

This domain offers little satisfaction to the nurse, because it is unsettling to discover that a "near miss" or a potential mistake could have been made. The competencies in this domain go unnoticed when things go well and mistakes are avoided; when things go wrong,

143

however, there are incident reports to be filed and the nurse is confronted with a sense of guilt over not catching the error regardless of its source. Yet the nurse is in the best position to safeguard and coordinate the patient's total care so that the multiple departments' efforts do not unwittingly conflict with one another.

I am puzzled when nurses vehemently maintain that they never veer from doctor's orders despite changes in patients' needs or conditions. It is not always possible or even warranted to consult a doctor for minor changes in orders. I am distressed when nurses rigidly follow doctor's orders for diet or other comfort measures when the order is clearly outdated and the patient's comfort is sacrificed to a ritualized chain of command. I agree that in the best of all worlds the doctor is advised of changes in the patient's condition, anticipates change, and writes flexible orders that allow nurses to use their judgment. But in the contingencies of everyday practice, the safe and compassionate nurse chooses reason over ritual, and reasoned, good judgment is usually respected.

Where good communication exists between doctors and nurses and collaborative interactions prevail, flexibility increases and the patient benefits. Where this communication style does not exist and rules are followed rigidly, patients frequently spend unneeded hours on liquid diets or, worse yet, wait needlessly for their "nothing by mouth" sentence to be removed. Some flexibility has been added to postoperative care by routine standing orders that can be changed according to the nurse's judgment of the patient's progress. Unit self-studies would be useful to document recurring delays in changes of doctor's orders, causing patients unnecessary discomfort. The outcome of such studies could be new agreements between physicians and nurses on the more common areas of difficulty.

10 | Organizational and Work-Role Competencies

     This domain, more than any other, is dependent on learning on the job. Increasingly, nursing schools are adding more managerial and leadership training to their programs because the nurse works predominantly in complex organizations. However, even principles taught by simulation and case study cannot capture the complexity of the organizational demands placed on the new nurse, who must learn the local, the particular, the contingent, and the historical in mastering management and leadership on a particular unit.

Many of the competencies (see box on page 147) discovered in this domain were observed under the worst constraints of understaffing. In keeping with the study's goals to identify competencies, the many probable deficits in care under these conditions were not documented, but it was clear that these nurses did not like doing what they called "emergency nursing." They were uncomfortable with the meagre knowledge they had about their patients and extremely dissatisfied with the fact that they often could do only too little and too late. There were no descriptions of "early warning"; only the obvious and most demanding needs were attended to. These nurses' dissatisfactions and coping strategies point to another obviously needed area of descriptive research: the documentation of care deficits under different organizational and staffing conditions.

Coordinating, Ordering, and Meeting Multiple Patient Needs and Requests: Setting Priorities

In interviewing pairs of beginning nurses and preceptors, one competency labeled as "organization" was invariably mentioned as a hurdle and a change in performance capability. These nurses — both the experienced and the neophytes — talked about the time when they responded to every request with almost equal intensity and speed. In terms of level of skill acquisition, this kind of response would occur during the novice and advanced beginner stages before the nurse had acquired a sense of salience — of perceiving that some things were more important than others. Upon observation it was notable that expert nurses had the ability to juggle and integrate multiple patient requests and care needs without losing important information or missing significant needs. In the first exemplar the transition from the advanced beginner stage to competency is evident.

EXEMPLAR I

New Nurse: In nursing school you have very few patients. And then I came on here and I still have few patients, but I didn't realize all the lifting and the time it took because I'd want to get... I don't know... I'd come here and I'd get all my sheets out

Domain: Organizational and Work-Role Competencies

Coordinating, Ordering, and Meeting Multiple Patient Needs and Requests: Setting Priorities

Building and Maintaining a Therapeutic Team to Provide Optimum Therapy

Coping with Staff Shortages and High Turnover:

Contingency planning

Anticipating and preventing periods of extreme work overload within a shift

Using and maintaining team spirit; gaining social support from other nurses

Maintaining a caring attitude toward patients even in absence of close and frequent contact

Maintaining a flexible stance toward patients, technology, and bureaucracy

and go pass them around and then somebody would want a glass of water or this and that and I used to just run, jump anytime a patient said anything. And that would just totally disorganize me. Because I was constantly running around. And I never got anything done. So I've learned to set priorities. Water is not really a priority as compared to a pain shot or getting everything passed out and saying, "Just a minute. I'll come back."

If you saw me in the beginning you would see me making a hundred trips up and down the hall with a very frustrated look on my face, almost in tears and never really accomplishing much of

147

anything. You would probably have to give me a lot of help. You would be watching somebody give me a lot of help. Now, I still have my moments, I mean everybody does where they are still unorganized, but AM care is done usually by ten and new medications are given right away, charting is done earlier, things run more smoothly. Now I feel more compassionate and more empathy for my patients.

Interviewer: Now, than you did when you first came?

New Nurse: Oh, yes. I was too worried about everything else to really look at my patients, to even care about them.

Interviewer: Now I'm sure that's typical and that's part of the process you go through. How could you attend? The patients become objects where you're having to coordinate so many things. Just moving up and down the hall so often can be difficult at first.

New Nurse: For awhile I wondered if I wanted to be a nurse. Because I didn't really care. It was just so hard for me to get my medications out and do all that, that I didn't even care. Now, I don't know. I really care about them. I feel like, I don't know what it was. I just walked in one day and felt like this was home. Everybody was in their beds and their places, and they all have real feelings, and I really wanted to get to know these people and see what they needed. And it feels good.

EXEMPLAR II

Participant Observation of an Expert Nurse's Performance: She seems to know what she wants to accomplish with each of them during the evening. She has encouraged liquids with Bob, who does look pale and dehydrated. She later does a fresh urine and finds that his sugar is now 5 plus, and remarks, "I don't know why he's spilling sugar like that." The other man in the room is to have eye surgery in the morning. She tells him that she will come in later and do some explaining about the surgery. She asks him if he wants anything to drink, and he tells her that he would like some tomato juice. She has him put his own eye drops in his left eye. He touches the sclera and she corrects him, telling him not to touch the eye when he puts the drops in. She talks to me in the hall telling me the plans and concerns about her patients. We then went into Sarah's room because Dr. A was there and wanted the nurse there when he talked with the patient and examined her. He wanted to ask the nurse questions. She told the doctor that Sarah was more alert this evening, perkier, and clearer.

The things that Ellen has in mind for her patients seem to be very integrated, of a whole piece of cloth. She remembers the tomato juice promised to the pre-op eye patient within good time, but after doing many other things. She was in Sarah's room and then in Jean's room, yet she did not forget the tomato juice. I mentioned this—"How did you remember the tomato juice? You seem to keep a lot in your head." She said, "You know, sometimes I'm amazed at how much I remember, and that I don't forget, but if I did have to do everything, one thing at a time, then I would just be running and would not have time to do everything. I would be making too many trips."

Summary Statement   This advanced competency is often more visible in its absence and thus may go un-noticed and unrewarded. Experienced nurses learn to organize, plan, and coordinate multiple patient needs and requests and to reshuffle their priorities in the midst of constant patient changes.

Building and Maintaining a Therapeutic Team to Provide Optimum Therapy

Every health team member with responsibility for a patient will assess that patient's potential for wellness. And for the therapy to be optimally effective, each person involved must present his or her perspective to the other team members. This exchange is an ongoing process, because the patient changes from time to time and because different relationships elicit different perspectives and therefore different possibilities for therapy.

Working as a team is crucial both for providing effective patient therapy and for maintaining morale among team members. Differences of opinion are inevitable and a necessary part of effective therapy. When disagreements lead to breaches among team members, though, efforts must be made to recreate the team.

EXEMPLAR I

A nurse describes the aftermath of a major confrontation between herself and a doctor over giving a patient EST (shock therapy):

We'd missed a really valuable step, and that was in getting the doctors involved in writing policy with us. Even though it's not as strong, some people would say rigid, as I would like, at least it's generally followed because it was passed by the psychiatric staff. . . what I think is that it's real important saying, "We're in this together, even if we're disagreeing."

EXEMPLAR II

Participant Observation: The nurse states that the team also includes the other shifts. An expert nurse emphasizes the importance of this extended notion of team and shows how it works with the example of her shift helping the earlier shift ventilate when there had been a suicide during the night, and by the example of doing extra work for a new admit at the end of her shift because of the chaos that naturally occurs at report time. But the team relationship must involve both give *and* take. Thus, when the team relationship among shifts is established, the next shift can be relied on to help out when the current shift can no longer cope.

Expert Nurse: Hopefully, you have a good enough relationship with the shift that's following that on those days when you just need to leave something, you can say, "I'm sorry, I really need to leave this. We've got to get out of here." And that's really nice when that's happening.

Finally, this skill includes the ability to recreate or rebuild the team after a breakdown.

Summary Statement The team building exemplars came primarily from an acute psychiatric setting; however, effective team effort and coordination between shifts and among team members are essential to any therapeutic environment – not only for continuity but also for the survival and health of the team members. Patient care is much too demanding and complex to be accomplished by any *one* team member.

It was evident that expert nurses recognize the team as an integral part of their own effectiveness as they are in the business world.

Coping with Staff Shortages and High Turnover

Intermittent shortages of nurses and high staff turnover saddle nurses with work overload and the additional stresses associated with working with temporary and inexperienced staff. When the data for this study were being collected, nurses were in short supply, although the situation would probably alter with economic downswings. These shifts in supply and demand will always be a factor in skilled nursing performance. Nursing care is demanding and stressful under the best of circumstances, but under these additional strains nurses must drastically alter their role performance and coping strategies. All six hospitals where these data were collected were experiencing staff shortages; only one private community hospital had an unusually low turnover rate.

But one inner-city, general, teaching hospital was suffering extreme staff shortages at the time of data collection. The turnover and staff shortage had reached a crisis and self-perpetuating level. There were noticeable differences in the content of the nurses' descriptions of their practice in this hospital. There, they talked only about patient care crises, near misses, and frank patient care failures. These were the situations where they thought that their interventions had made a positive difference, although they seldom felt that they were able to offer enough at the right time. When asked if there were less crisis-oriented situations that stood out in their minds, they described the time pressure involved in accomplishing just the *necessary* patient care tasks. For one nurse to administer all the intravenous therapy to some 23 patients left that nurse with precious little time to attend to other patient care needs. One nurse summed it up this way: "You shortcut. You learn all the shortcuts. You learn all the priorities and you do emergency nursing."

What happens to the nursing role under these conditions? In addition to the absence of descriptions of non-crisis-oriented patient care situations, nurses in this hospital did not talk about the patients as persons in their interviews. There were few indications of who the patients were, what their illnesses interrupted, or how the patients interpreted their illnesses. This was quite different from the small group and individual interviews conducted in the other hospitals. In the third interview session the nurses were asked about this omission. Their responses were telling.

Interviewer: One of the things that I haven't heard you talk about so far is your relationship with patients.

Nurse I: It really doesn't exist. You don't have an opportunity to develop any sort of human relationship with the patients because you are so busy. We have some very, very sick patients.

Staff Development Nurse: But when I go to the floor, I see gifts and cards and lot of things that say, "Thanks, I don't know what I would have done without you."

Nurse I: Yes, that's there because the LVNs are with the patients. They make the human connection all the time, right? But I don't; I'm removed.

These nurses cope with this role deprivation by fostering a caring attitude even when they have little time for their normal ways of delivering care.

The continual strain of work overload, coping with temporary staff, and orienting new staff members understandably perpetuates the high turnover. But in addition to this major source of dissatisfaction, other important sources of work satisfaction are also missing. These nurses cope with their jobs primarily by responding to the challenge of the situation. But they frequently end up feeling that they have offered too little, too late. Thus, two important sources of satisfaction are missing: the human connection, and the sense of competency and accomplishment that comes from knowing that you have been able to offer what you had to offer *when* it was needed. The working environment of these nurses has ceased to be a self-sustaining system.

The nurses pointed out that they felt as if they had little time for reflection, so their own learning and growth had stopped. Most of their reflection was done at home, where they were not able to check out or pursue their hunches. Indeed, one could speculate that they talked about only crisis-oriented incidents, because these were the only incidents that they remembered. With their information overload, only these events stood out for retelling. Needless to say, these nurses found it difficult to feel proud of their accomplishments because to do so would have been to sanction their working conditions. They called what they were doing "emergency nursing" and hoped they could hold out until some improvements were made.

Contingency Planning. Working under a heavy workload, the nurse has to rapidly assess the most crucial patient care and surveillance needs: read the clinical situation, set priorities, and shift them frequently. Routine standards, procedures, and guidelines must be continually evaluated in the context of multiple needs. It is a constant process of triage. Nurses report that some priorities are standard: for example, dangerous vital sign readings, medical and surgical emergencies such as shock, high fevers, saturated dressings, I.V. medications running dry, piggyback I.V. medications. But even these high priorities get shifted around during a patient crisis on the unit.

EXEMPLAR I

Expert Nurse: It's just that the pace is so fast. On days the pace is fast, and you're moving and going so many different places that we're overwhelmed. We have to pass meds, we have to team lead, we have to see if so and so is doing her job and how did she do that dressing. Did she pack it properly? You know, that's just too much.

EXEMPLAR II

Interviewer: So it becomes sort of—given the context and given the circumstances—how do you do as well as you do? How do you deliver an acceptable level of care?

Nurse 1: You do emergency nursing.

Nurse 2: Find out what is most needed.

Nurse 3: Prioritize right at the beginning of the shift.

Nurse 4: You must have a routine. You must have some sort of organization. The one thing that is really hard on the floor is when you have an emergency and you have to pull people from way down the hall, get all the help together to move this bed out of the room. Like Ellen helped me one day with a patient who was on a respirator and there was no bed in the ICU. And so Ellen stayed over. I got everybody on the whole floor. We moved the bed, got the patient intubated. We got the respirator in there, and she stayed and helped.

Nurse 1: And then you're behind the entire night?

Nurse 4: No, I finally caught up *because the nurse who was taking care of him knew what to do.* But it's very difficult in a crisis situation on the floor when you've got to go down the hall to pull this person, pull that person, to get it all together.

These nurses also provided examples of when they simply could not regroup their forces and do contingency planning. For example, there was one nurse for 40 acutely ill patients, and a patient had a cardiac arrest at the beginning of the shift. The situation defied any kind of contingency planning.

Anticipating and Preventing Periods of Extreme Work Overload Within a Shift.   In acute care situations there is some ability to smooth out the work overload within a shift. But particular periods during a shift are chronically overloaded – for example, during change of shift. Experienced nurses become adept at anticipating and avoiding additional demands during the critical periods of high demand and overload.

EXEMPLAR

Expert Nurse: I've learned to handle the MICU transferring people because they usually wait until quarter 'til three or 3:00 to transfer a patient. So I get the nurses to give me a report before that time, because I know they're going to transfer at 3:00. So then I'll have time to listen to them. Or I'll go inside there and give report and then it doesn't matter what time they bring a patient out then, if I already have the report. This prevents the interruption while I'm trying to do something else.

Using and Maintaining Team Spirit: Gaining Social Support from Other Nurses.   Working under conditions in which each nurse has a high patient load requires that individuals find ways of being supported, even when others cannot always be there to help out. The sense of being "under fire" together generates a sense of camaraderie that cannot be duplicated under other circumstances.

EXEMPLAR

A patient had a blocked tracheostomy tube and there was no suction machine—even more crucial, there were no tweezers.

> *Nurse:* Well, one thing that was really good was that the MICU nurses responded so well. I had their sympathy and their empathy. And they were willing to stop whatever they were doing to come out and help me with this.

Maintaining a Caring Attitude Toward Patients Even in Absence of Close and Frequent Contact. When a single nurse has anywhere from 20 to 40 patients under her care and is the only R.N. on her team, she or he will not have the time to have close personal contact with patients. But the fact that many patients are either chronic (readmitted often), or so acute that their stay is prolonged enables the nurse to get to know and care personally about the outcome of these patients' illnesses.

EXEMPLAR I

> *Interviewer:* This is something that's always really interesting. You seem to recognize patients from different units. How does this happen?
>
> *Nurse 1:* Well, see, we had him before.
>
> *Nurse 2:* We had him up on 5th.
>
> *Nurse 3:* And he'd always come up to visit us.

Nurse 4: What's really sad is when one of these patients that travels around dies.

Nurse 2: Yeah.

Nurse 3: Everybody gets word of it.

Nurse 1: That's what we're afraid of with Jim . . .

EXEMPLAR II

Interviewer: It's hard for me to imagine how you stay connected. How do you keep this patient human for yourself? How do you work with her? Could you tell me anything about that?

Nurse 1: Well, Linda happens to be a very human person, I mean, she's just very talkative and expressive. I mean, it's very hard to forget all of Linda, even when you're working on one of her parts.

Nurse 2: She reminds you.

Interviewer: Say more about that. Say more about Linda. I mean how does she . . . I suspect that she does things to help you work with her perhaps. And maybe you could say something about that.

Nurse 1: She has a good outlook on life. I don't know. Even though she knows the prospect is very poor for her, she seems to think she is going to get better and she has confidence in her doctor that when you talk to her she knows. She thinks positive and she gives you this positive attitude. Even though you know she's not going to get any better. So we just keep going on and doing things and we hope, like her, that she will get better.

Maintaining a Flexible Stance Toward Patients, Technology, and Bureaucracy. Experienced nurses see their work in terms of goals. But to attain goals in a less than perfect world, they develop a flexible stance that allows them to accept idiosyncratic patient behavior, find technological substitutes in emergencies, and get around others' inflexible behavior.

EXEMPLAR I

Field Notes: The nurses talked about several patients who came up to their units to select their beds *before* they went to the admitting office. The two patients being described had long-term illnesses. The nurses went on to talk about the exceptions and accommodations now made by the unit for these patients, as the staff has learned their preferences and their ways of coping with their illnesses. They also talked about their dreading to see these patients lose ground in their fight with their serious illnesses.

EXEMPLAR II

An expert nurse describes how she clamped a chest tube when no clamps were available:

Of course there was no clamp. And it was 4:20. I was the only person out on the floor. The other people had gone in to their report. All of them. So I was the only other person out there except for these other souls from I don't know where. And there weren't any clamps. So I just grabbed it and held it. Somebody found a rubber band, and we put a rubber band around it. Then I ran out and called CSR and I said, "Send a clamp up." And they did. I couldn't believe it. They sent one up and I clamped it off.

EXEMPLAR III

Field Notes: Hospital policy prohibits drawing of blood, doing EKGs, administering skin tests, and insertion of I.V.s by nurses in their teaching hospital. In tight situations nurses work around these policies simply because the situation calls for immediate action. In other cases they protest because it is inconvenient to have to coordinate with another department to get the particular prohibited procedure done. Thus, these performances that are commonly done by nurses are done despite hospital policy when the situation warrants.

Summary Statement Acute staff shortages and work overload create a crisis-ridden organizational climate. Maximum flexibility is required to cope with the constraints and shortages, so nurses find ways to work as flexibly as possible within the constraints of their circumstances.

Summary and Conclusions

These competencies point out the demanding and complex nature of the nursing role in the hospital setting. Competencies associated with team building require social integration before the new entrant can actually be skilled in building and maintaining a therapeutic team. To provide continuity and safe care around the clock takes coordination and teamwork.

Our cultural bias is to prefer the individualistic, autonomous aspects of any work role, and nursing has sought to decrease the fragmentation of care and increase the accountability and visibility of the nurse through the introduction of primary nursing. But regardless of the efforts to give individual nurses the authority and autonomy that will match their actual responsibilities, nurses will continue to need exquisite organizational and work role skills.

The next two chapters present the broader implications of the seven domains of nursing care for nursing research and nursing practice, as well as for career development and nursing education.

11 | Implications for Research and Clinical Practice

It is a tribute to the richness of nursing practice that each of the competencies presented in the seven domains of nursing practice yields multiple implications for research, clinical practice, career development, and education. I will discuss the first two in this chapter.

Involvement versus Distance

Each domain and exemplar raise possible research questions. I separated the "helping role" from the "teaching-coaching function," for instance, even though they can both be considered helping behaviors, because of the richness of these two domains and because the caring exhibited in the helping domain is dictinct from teaching and also from what is typically described as "therapeutic." The word "therapeutic" has inherited meaning from the psychoanalytic perspective that defines the helper as one who establishes "distance" as a part of the "professional" relationship. These "helping" nurses, however, repeatedly described a committed, involved relationship. They said things like: "We had become friends." "We really knew each other well by this time, and I understood the family and the patient." "I thought of him as my grandfather, and I cared about what was happening to him."

During these interviews, I thought of all my nursing courses where I had been warned not to become "too involved." And I asked how the nurses managed this business of being involved and yet having to subject the patient to painful procedures. I developed a hypothesis from the answers I received that remains untested. I hypothesized that by *being* involved, these nurses were more fully able to draw on their own coping resources and the resources offered by the patient, family, and the situation. I suspect that the distancing techniques dimly protect nurses from the pain in the situation, but they also prevent them from taking advantage of the resources and possibilities that come through engagement and participation in the patients' and families' meanings and ways of coping.

A few nurses stood out as less involved, as purposely choosing to distance themselves, but they were in the minority, as reflected in the exemplars. This opens up the possibility of some provocative research. The Dreyfus model of skill acquisition would predict that a certain level of commitment and involvement is necessary for a sense of salience to develop. A "distanced" observer is less likely to notice subtle changes in patients. Thus, a certain level of commitment and involvement is necessary for expert performance. Nurses' actual practices and the demonstrations of expertise in this study challenge some of our formal and informal ideology about maintaining distance from patients.

| Nurse–Patient Relationships

As a researcher currently taking courses in graduate psychology, I recognized that the helping language of the nurse was distinct from that of other health care providers. This uniqueness calls for more exploration, more descriptive research. By their very position, nurses are asked different questions and looked to for different kinds of help than other professionals. In the course of the participant observations, for example, I watched nurses assisting patients with ileostomy and colostomy bag and dressing changes. If the patient was hospitalized for a surgical revision and had been managing at home, the discussion quickly moved to questions about how the patient was managing at home. "Are you getting dressed and out in the morning?" The questions were specific, focusing on common issues in home management, and moved quite naturally to explore feelings of acceptance and evidence of adjustment.

The questions asked by these nurses came from their discussions with many patients on the specific daily coping issues and strategies. One patient, referred to earlier, even asked a nurse during a preoperative mastectomy teaching session if the nurse had had a mastectomy, because her manner was so accepting and so knowledgeable about the passages the patient could expect after surgery. In this manner, nurses as coaches did not place themselves, nor did their patients place them, outside the realm of possibly experiencing the same illnesses.

When I asked nurses about this, they said that it was important for them to come to terms in some personal way with what the patient was confronting before they became good at working with patients with particular illnesses. The exemplars in both the helping and coaching domains offer clues to uncharted knowledge about the unique nurse–patient relationship that waits to be uncovered through clinical ethnographies in existing clinical practice.

Since it is through informal learning that nurses learn ways of coping and possibilities inherent in illness and recovery trajectories, it makes sense that systematic nursing research focused on the phenomenology of recovery would add to the nurse's knowledge and skill as a coach. Such studies would have to go beyond mere descriptions of the information that patients want to know. They would have to be clinical ethnographies of recovery trajectories that would capture the issues, adaptive demands, fears, conflicts, and capabilities across different patients with different personal and situational characteristics.

Early Warning Signals

The diagnostic and patient monitoring function of the nurse has increased with increasing acuity levels and more sophisticated treatment regimens that have narrow margins of therapeutic safety. The nurse perceiving early warning signals is crucial in intensive care units and even more crucial on the intermediate care units where automated telemetry is not routinely used. The phenomenon of early perceptual recognition of patient changes needs to be more extensively studied to clarify what facilitates the development of this skill and how widespread is the impact of the nurse's early warning on the patient's recovery.

Educators have not attended sufficiently to the difference between being able to recognize a medical problem, being able to document it, and being able to present a defensible case that will get an appropriate physician response. Doing well in one aspect does not guarantee success in the other two. Nurses talked about the importance of gaining credibility with physicians, so that a correct early warning would increase the likelihood that the physician would take their vague early concerns more seriously in the future. On the other hand, it might be difficult to overcome the reputation of being an alarmist. To improve early recognition skills, nurses could keep a record of their own early warnings to determine when they overlooked a change in patient status or when they were overreacting.

Or else a unit might increase its credibility through self-study. Each nursing unit probably has its own predictable and repeated communication breakdowns with physicians, and a simple recording of problems could offer surprisingly simple solutions. Quality assurance studies might incorporate a study of nurse presentation of information and physician response based on that information. The problems presented in the exemplars illustrate that, despite much professional attention to the traditional nurse–physician communication problem, these problems are still at the forefront of many difficulties.

The diagnostic and monitoring domain illustrates the rapid changes in patients and the need for nurses to develop ways to cope with these changes. By studying how expert nurses manage to cope, we can learn new ways to teach students. For example, nurses could be taught how to give a "forward looking" report. Observing advance preparations, the expert nurse can uncover sets and assumptions that hold clinical knowledge.

The nurse's in-depth knowledge about a particular patient population offers the researcher much information for systematic study of stress and coping patterns within and between different illnesses. Since Stotland (1969) has demonstrated that hopelessness is contagious, and since nurses informally assess a patient's potential for wellness, this area of clinical knowledge can be laden with wisdom as well as with misperception. Both the wisdom and the misperceptions deserve study.

Outside the Boundaries of Nursing

Nurses are expected to manage rapidly changing situations until the physician arrives, but since this puts the nurse outside the usual boundaries of nursing practice, this skilled area is not formally acknowledged or well studied. Yet it is the nurse who calls for and coordinates multiple members of the health care team, whether it be by calling the physician or by calling a code blue. It is curious that we have conducted no studies in nursing about the rapid decison making required for calling a code blue, despite the fact that nurses must make split-second decisions about whether the problem is a simple faint, an artifact of telemetry, or the beginning of a catastrophic problem.

Unfortunately, some nurses may read these exemplars and say: "But this is not nursing!" While managing life-threatening emergencies in the absence of a physician is not the planned, formal role of the nurse, it is required of the nurse in actual practice, and more documentation and legitimization of this function would probably improve the nurse's preparation for it. I was struck that nurses do not seek the opportunity to function in this role, nor do they feel rewarded for outstanding performance in the face of limited resources and great odds. Usually they feel sad because the system has not worked as it should. This domain offers important avenues for further research. Perhaps extensive documentation of this frequent responsibility of the nurse would bring the legitimization that would improve both the performance and coping resources of the nurse and the system.

Monitoring and Organizational Skills

Some of the domains of nursing practice described in this book have not been sufficiently legitimized, but that is not the case with the domain of administration and monitoring of therapeutic regimens. Nurses expect to administer and monitor highly complicated treatments. Much time is spent in nursing education or in the literature in describing new procedures, but little attention is given to the high level of skill necessary to carry out these procedures with minimal pain and risk. Once acquired, these skills may seem simple or even unimportant. But we have much to learn from nurses who are skilled at weaning patients from antiarrhythmia drugs or vasopressors. Descriptive knowledge of these skills would open up new areas for research and offer ways to improve clinical practice. We are limited only by skilled nurses' taking for granted the wisdom they have acquired.

Lewis Thomas (1983) describes the nurse as the glue that keeps the complicated system of hospital care together. Monitoring and ensuring the quality of care delivered by all health team members, along with expert organizational and work role skills, make up this invisible glue that keeps the system working. Because this is a taken-for-granted function of nurses, they themselves fail to recognize its importance. Like it or not, the organizational resources, constraints, and demands set limits and create options for skilled nursing practice. Therefore, the context – the organizational setting of nursing – cannot be excluded or considered an extraneous variable, as it both creates and is created by the nurse's participation in it. We have much to learn by studying the variation in nursing practices that can be accounted for by specific organizational characteristics. We need more studies that describe the nurse–patient relationship in a variety of organizational conditions.

The Phenomenon of Caring

There are more general conclusions to draw from these exemplars of excellent nursing practice. They point to the central role of caring, of a committed, involved stance in nursing practice. By including the context we are also able to talk about the quality of the caring, because caring is relational. By describing different kinds of caring in different kinds of contexts, we begin to understand the role of caring in healing and recovery. We do violence to caring when we separate in our practice the distinctions we are able to make conceptually between the "instrumental role" and the "expressive" role (Skipper, 1965).

The expert nurse melds these two roles. Consider, for example, the patient who pointed to her exquisitely designed and technically sophisticated dry dressing and commented with a note of hopefulness instead of the despair expressed only hours before: "Look at this dressing – isn't it a work of art?" (see p. 131). The changing of the dressing was, all at the same time, technical, expressive, and transformative. The patient's relationship to her wound and her expectations for her care had changed in the transaction.

One way to separate the instrumental and expressive aspects of nursing is to relegate caring to the art of nursing. But once we consider caring as artful (although I agree that it is), we risk ignoring caring as a subject of scholarly inquiry. As a result, both our practice and theory will suffer. This is a real danger for a profession whose central aim is care. To examine "care," we cannot rely on purely quantitative, experimental measurements based on the natural science model. Nursing is a human science, conducted by self-interpreting subjects (researchers) who are studying self-interpreting subjects (participants) who *both* may change as a result of an investigation (Heidegger, 1962; Palmer, 1969; Taylor, 1971; Bourdieu, 1977). Caring cannot be controlled or coerced; it can only be understood and facilitated. Caring is embedded in personal and cultural meanings and commitments (Wrubel, Benner & Lazarus, 1981; Benner, in press). Therefore, the strategies for studying it must take into account meanings and commitments.

Bellah (1982) contrasts investigations that are "communicative, practical, and ethical rather than manipulative, technological, and scientific" (if scientific is understood only in the model of the natural sciences). He states:

> I am suggesting that we reverse the priorities between technical and practical interests, between techne and praxis, between control and action. The purpose of practice is not to produce or control anything but to discover through mutual discussion and reflection between free citizens the most appropriate ways, under present conditions, of living the ethically good life. To that end technological knowledge may be helpful, provided that it is

171

used in the context of a practical (that is, ethical and political) knowledge that takes precedence over it (p. 36).

Although Bellah is speaking to sociologists, politicians, and ethicists, his advice is equally appropriate for nursing—an applied discipline that cannot "care" without considering the ethics and meanings involved in the practices of caring.

12 | Implications for Career Development and Education

As the preceding chapters have made evident, the Dreyfus Model of Skill Acquisition, applied to nursing, demonstrates the progression of expertise that can result from experience. The interpretive approach that has been used here to describe nursing practice demonstrates the level of risk and discretionary judgment currently exercised by expert nurses. Both the model and the approach illustrate the need for a systematic approach to career development in hospital nursing practice. Nursing management strategies must take into consideration the current level of responsibility, knowledge, and clinical judgment exercised by the expert nurse practicing in the hospital. At present, there is a recognition lag and consequently a mismanagement of highly skilled nurses.

Further, the Dreyfus model provides a rationale for the development of a career ladder of promotion, because it predicts the kinds of expertise and knowledge that are gained by experience. We have increasingly clarified the gains made by continuing education and advanced degrees in nursing, but little attention has been given to what can be learned from clinical experience. Both the Dreyfus model and the interpretive approach to describing nursing practice presented here demonstrate the latter kind of learning.

Career Development

Both environmental and internal changes in nursing call for increased attention to career development and retention of nurses working in positions of direct patient care. With advances in health and medical care, the role and responsibilities of nursing have increased. In fact, the role and functions of clinical nursing in acute care settings have grown so complex that it is no longer possible to standardize or routinize much of what the nurse does. Patient acuity levels have increased, and the numbers of diagnostic and treatment interventions available have increased. Indeed, the major rationale for hospitalization today is the need for expert nursing care. The current complexity of nursing makes interchangeabilty and easy replacement of nurses expensive and not conducive to quality care. Furthermore, in this equal rights era, women plan for and expect careers with progressive advancement rather than intermittent, disconnected jobs. There is a concerted effort to decrease sex segregation in nursing by increased recruitment of men into the profession.

One further change supports the need for increased tenure and experience for nurses in hospital settings. That change is a shift to a more holistic approach to the understanding of disease (Cassell, 1976; Bursztajn, Feinbloom, Hamm, & Brodsky, 1981; Cousins, 1983). The attention to the whole patient and the effects of stress and coping on the course of an illness — areas traditionally emphasized by nurses—are more and more recognized as critical variables in patient recovery. Similarly, relational, interpretive, and coaching functions of nurses are increasingly recognized as central to patient recovery and health promotion (see Chapters 4 and 5). But holistic patient care requires experience and continuity in nursing care delivery. Shorter hospital stays have also increased the need for continuity and highly experienced nursing care, since short stays allow little or no time for stable periods of recuperation. In the past, longer hospital stays lent themselves to routinization and delegation of care to other personnel after the acute stages were past.

In an effort to minimize the effects of high turnover in nursing, nurse managers have attempted to standardize and routinize nursing practice where possible. Written guidelines, policies, and procedures, as a form of explicit culture, have proliferated in nursing (Gordon, p. 191) to fill in the knowledge gaps of the steady stream of new staff nurses. Standards and policies have also proliferated to meet the legal requirements for the delegation of tasks to nurses by physician and hospital policies. Thus, there has been excessive formalization of hospital nursing despite the nurse's increasing discretionary responsibility for patient welfare.

At the same time, few incentives or rewards for long-term careers in hospital nursing have been offered. To advance in pay, status, and quality of work life, nurses have switched careers or chosen administrative positions, teaching, or some form of community health nursing over long-term positions in direct patient care in hospitals. This tradition of short-term hospital employment has been further entrenched by the common view that nursing as a woman's profession can not be expected to promote long-term career positions. As "woman's work," nursing has traditionally been considered intermittent and short-term. Therefore, few strategies and structures in hospital personnel management have been geared to retaining the experienced nurse clinician in positions of direct patient care.

Nursing is an emerging profession — one that is ill-equipped to reward and recognize excellence in hospital nursing practice. Most administrative and managerial resources have been spent in managing the high turnover. However, the very tactics for managing high turnover militate against career development and the enhancement of expertise. Today's nurse is a professional clinician — a knowledgeable worker — whose role complexity and responsibility require long-term, continuing development. This chapter offers a framework for clinical knowledge development in hospital nursing practice, for career development in positions of direct patient care, and for management practices designed to reward and retain excellent clinical nurses at the patient's bedside.

Nursing is faced with two conflicting mandates: (1) to individualize patient care, and (2) to minimize errors through maintaining minimal standards of patient care (e.g., all patients must have siderails up on their beds at night.) Thus the standards, rules, and guidelines geared to achieve an acceptable standard of care can at the same time prevent the individualization of that care. The research reported here demonstrates that the expert nurse can interpret particular situations and make the necessary exceptions and alterations in the rules in order to individualize patient care; the knowledge embedded in the expert's clinical practice transcends norms and expected procedures. In other words, even "high" standards of care can be surpassed by expertise and generosity.

176

The danger, however, is that the findings of this study might be misunderstood as one more way of standardizing practice and that the 31 competencies described here will be mistaken for new standards to be legislated. Such a misapplication would be unfortunate because expertise cannot be legislated or standardized although it can be facilitated, recognized, and rewarded. It cannot be standardized, since expertise in a situation always involves an accurate interpretation of specific responses to a specific situation. It *always* involves discretionary judgment and *often* risk. In fact, if one tries to decontextualize and standardize the "essential features" of expert human decision making, the result is, at most, a minimal level of competency, similar to what can be achieved through systems analysis and computer programs (Dreyfus, 1979; Dreyfus, 1982; Dreyfus & Dreyfus, in press).

It must be clarified that the exemplars of expert practice presented in the preceding chapters are not intended to be additional or new standards of practice; instead, they are a representative sample of current clinical nursing practice in hospitals. Any attempt to extract their "essential features" and make them into guidelines is not likely to succeed. For example, expert nurses discontinue treatments that they judge irrelevant or harmful as a result of changes in the patient's condition or competing patient needs. Guidelines can be extracted for these exceptions, but they will never replace the expert's grasp of the specific situation. Therefore, guidelines for exceptions may be less intelligent than the original rule, order, or guideline that is being altered. There is no higher court than the expert's reading of a *particular* situation.

The nurse clinician is confronted with complex and ambiguous patient care situations. Sometimes decisions are made to meet one important patient care need at the expense of another important need. Not even expertise can rid the clinician of the uncertainty inherent in clinical practice. Difficult choices are made based on the best judgment in the particular situation. This is called "setting priorities," but the language of priority setting betrays the complexity and residual uncertainty of the choices. This research calls for expanding the ways of describing and thinking about nursing expertise and about nursing practice itself.

Experience, as it is used here, does not necessarily refer to longevity or length of time in a position; rather, it refers to a very active process of refining and changing preconceived theories, notions, and ideas when confronted with actual situations. This model assumes that all practical situations are far more complex than can be described by formal models, theories, and textbook descriptions. In encountering clinical situations with their many nuances, qualitative differences, and confounding problems, clinicians gain a different understanding of theory or preconceived notions. Theory is crucial to forming the right questions to ask in a clinical situation; theory tells the practitioner where to look for problems and how to anticipate care needs. But there is always more to a situation than the theory predicts. It is this learning about the exceptions and shades of meaning that only concrete experience can provide.

In the Dreyfus model, skilled performance is defined situationally rather than as a talent or trait that transcends all situations. Therefore, this model would predict that a nurse might perform at an expert level (given the innate ability and adequate educational preparation) in a clinical situation where she or he (1) is highly experienced, (2) is motivated to perform well, and (3) has the usual resources and constraints associated with that situation. But this same nurse might perform at various levels of skill if these conditions were different. Since nurses do not control the patients in their caseload, and since novel and unusual clinical situations will always occur in clinical practice, one can reasonably expect a nurse to perform at the expert level, for example, in familiar situations and at the competent or even advanced beginner level in less familiar ones. Thus, this model does not support certifying nurses as *novice, competent,* or *expert* for all situations.

Organizational support structures might be more important to career development than the particular written policy and salary structure developed. Organizational supports for career development indicated by this research include opportunities and structures for clinical specialization, staffing stability, and the legitimization of increased discretionary decision making for the expert.

Clinical Specialization

The situational nature of skilled performance predicted by the Dreyfus model is borne out in the interviews and observations of nursing practice. The same nurse typically describes critical incidents illustrative of several levels of skilled performance. For example, a nurse who was expert in intensive coronary care found it difficult to perform even at the competent level on an intermediate care surgical unit. And nurses working on units with extremely high staff turnover simply did not have circumstances under which they could acquire expertise. Moreover, clinical expertise turns out to be highly influenced by experience with similar patient populations. This supports clinical specialization and a structure of clinical preceptors to teach the beginning nurse or the experienced nurse who transfers to a new unit. This is particularly important since the nurse's monitoring and assessment function requires graded qualitative distinctions that can be made only by someone who has an experiential basis for comparing similar and dissimilar cases.

The complex decision making illustrated in the competencies described in the domains, "The Diagnostic and Patient Monitoring Function of the Nurse"; "Effective Management of Rapidly Changing Situations"; and "Monitoring and Ensuring the Quality of Health Care Practices," calls for experienced nurses. They also require ongoing clinical teaching at the unit level. This kind of teaching is difficult to plan, because it requires the clinical situation at hand for instruction. Qualitative distinctions can be pointed out only when the clinical situation permits, and by an expert clinician who recognizes subtle clinical changes.

Clinical specialization with particular types of patients is also extremely important to the acquisition of competencies in the "Teaching–Coaching Function" and the "Helping Role" domains of nursing. Nurses acquire ways of understanding, interpreting, and coping with illnesses by taking care of many different patients with a range of comparable adjustment and coping demands. Flexibility and wisdom are gained from working with patients throughout all phases of their illness. A nurse who has not actually seen a range of deviations from normal will have difficulty in recognizing them and in teaching the patient what to expect.

Staff Development Programs

As indicated above, staff development on the unit level makes it feasible to compare similarities and differences in many clinical situations. Currently, staff development departments place great emphasis on teaching isolated skills and procedures. This research indicates that increased attention should be given to demonstrating more advanced clinical judgments.

Staff development programs need to promote clinical knowledge development so that each nurse learns from clinical experience. Strategies for clinical knowledge development have been described elsewhere (Benner & Wrubel, 1982) and will only be highlighted here. An important first step, though, is for nurses to develop consensus in relation to their clinical descriptive language. This is done increasingly in nursing rounds, but can be enhanced by systematic strategies for documenting and comparing clinical judgments and clinical language.

Nurses at the proficient and expert levels can benefit from exchanges, clinical case studies, and opportunities to conduct and participate in research on clinical problems. Currently, very few staff education programs are geared to the needs of nurses at these levels. Increased effort in this area would improve the quality of patient care and serve as a retention strategy for highly skilled nurses. Nurses need to keep clinical records of their "early warnings" and their paradigm cases in order to enhance and document their clinical learning. Such clinical record keeping would provide a rich background for research.

This model suggests different instructional strategies for each level of skill acquisition, as discussed in Chapter 2. It predicts that problem approach is similar within the same level of skill acquisition — more so within the first three levels than the last two. Since there is a qualitative difference between the competent level and higher levels (proficient and expert), a competent nurse might be the most suitable preceptor for the advanced beginner — that is, the newly graduated nurse; an instructor closer to the learner's skill level may be more aware of the learner's readiness than a nurse at a more advanced skill level. This has not been tested, but it is a provocative hypothesis. By the same reasoning, the competent nurse would benefit from clinical precepting by nurses at the proficient and expert levels.

Staffing Stability

This model predicts that the most skilled performance will be attained in situations where there is opportunity to gain comparable experience and develop a shared language with clinical colleagues. A clinical promotion ladder has been suggested as a retention strategy, along with improved staff development programs for the experienced nurse. Nursing management must strive for structures that foster stability in order to maximize expert clinical performance. Nurses have too frequently been seen as interchangeable — a perspective that is challenged by this study. Staffing strategies should be geared to staff units so that nurses who are expert with the particular patient population are available for consultation at all times.

Evaluation Strategies

Current evaluation strategies typically use context-free competencies and enabling skills as standards of performance. Therefore, only attributes and aspects of the situation are considered, and usually the person's ability to recognize and assess patient care attributes and aspects is measured. The ability to judge the relative importance of aspects and attributes (i.e., salience) is overlooked in this process. This model would predict that only the beginning and competent levels of practice can be evaluated in terms of context-free attributes and aspects. More holistic and qualitative strategies are required to judge performance at the advanced levels of skill acquisition.

One hospital participating in this research uses narrative descriptions of critical incidents that demonstrate expertise as one document in the peer review process for advancement to a Clinical Nurse III level (see Huntsman, Epilogue, p. 244). Nurses are asked to describe and document patient care situations where their interventions made a difference in patient outcomes. The narrative approach allows for description of the content and meanings surrounding the incident as well as the structure and process involved.

Legitimizing Advanced Levels of Practice

Most policies and procedures are designed to ensure safe care when it is delivered by the minimally competent nurse. There is little formal acknowledgement or legitimization of increased discretionary judgment at advanced levels of proficiency. Thus, these higher levels of performance become informally expected, but without reward or sanction. Formal recognition of advanced discretionary decision making with clinical promotion legitimizes promotion on the basis of skill rather than longevity. Formal sanction also reduces the considerable amount of role strain and confusion asso-

183

ciated with unacknowledged responsibility. Only when ladders of clinical promotion match and reflect increased levels of proficiency will they serve as a basis for real career development.

| Nursing Education

The descriptions here of the scope of nursing practice, the amount of discretionary judgment called for, and the risks inherent in poor judgment indicate that strong educational preparation in the biological and psycho-social sciences and in nursing arts and science is the necessary base for advanced skill acquisition, because this knowledge provides the basis for safe care and gives the most advantageous position for gaining a sense of salience. Expertise takes time to develop, and it is neither cost-effective nor practical to try to "teach" it in formal educational programs. While the Dreyfus model outlines the process of advancement from novice to expert based on experience, the model assumes that theory and principles allow the practitioner safe and efficient access to clinical learning, provide the background knowledge that enables the clinician to ask the right questions and look for the correct problems. The person with limited background knowledge will lack the tools needed to learn from experience. Also, the scope of practice will be limited by the background knowledge the nurse brings to the clinical situation.

Clinical Specialization

Educational programs must prepare the nurse to function eventually at the advanced levels described here. In fact, such descriptions of actual nursing practice can

184

provide a basis for realistic curriculum planning (see Fenton, Epilogue). However, it is not economically feasible to prepare the new nurse at advanced levels of skill acquisition in more than one clinical area, since many clinical cases over time are necessary to acquire a sufficient base for advanced clinical judgment. Schools of nursing attempt to be efficient while extending the scope and depth of their students' educational experiences. But this research suggests that early clinical specialization in one area might be extremely advantageous in that it would give students an opportunity to learn about the process of acquiring advanced clinical knowledge.

Currently, nurses graduate with little understanding of the strategies for clinical skill acquisition beyond the advanced beginner or competent levels. Therefore, they have a secondary ignorance: they do not know what they do not know, and they have a limited understanding of how to go about learning it. Acquiring advanced levels of skill in one specialty area would teach the student what is involved in acquiring advanced skills in general. The goal of educational programs, of course, is to provide a broad base of clinical theory and skill that will provide the nurse with maximum flexibility and scope of practice after graduation. Thus the particular specialty offered in the school may not be the nurse's eventual choice, but the process of specialization could serve new nurses by offering them guidelines for acquiring a second specialty. The risk is that early specialization could limit the nurse's career flexibility.

Clinical Instruction

Nurse educators have grappled with the difficult problem of maintaining their clinical, teaching, and research expertise without any systematic structures for joint clinical and educational appointments. The findings of this research support clinical instruction from instructors at the advanced levels of skill acquisition for the advanced student. Probably it is not necessary for instructors of the novice to be able to perform clinically at the advanced levels. They need to be expert, however, at making visible the explicit guidelines and principles that will get the novice into the clinical situation in a safe and efficient way. But as the students advance in clinical specialization, they need teachers who can themselves demonstrate advanced levels of clinical judgment. Expert clinicians in the clinical setting can augment clinical instruction by pointing up patient problems that are unusual and by illustrating what is normally expected. This kind of clinical comparison process based upon clinical situations at hand requires joint effort between the preceptor on the patient care unit and the nurse educator.

Clinical Internships and Precepting

The Dreyfus model provides the concepts needed to differentiate between what can be taught by precept and what must be learned experientially from comparison of similar and dissimilar cases. New nurses are usually at the advanced beginner levels in most clinical areas, so clinical experts are needed on the patient care unit level to provide on-the-spot clinical teaching. This means that current efforts at providing clinical preceptors for neophyte nurses should be strengthened. New nurses should be prepared for the kinds of additional clinical judgment skills they will eventually need to acquire. Advanced planning for this stage in their clinical development will do much to help them cope with the deliberation (and the uncertainty) inherent in gaining proficiency.

This model also forecasts some of the difficulty they will have in learning from the expert. Too often the expert's difficulty in making all that he or she knows explicit is misunderstood by the beginner. An intellectual appreciation of the difficulty in conveying qualitative, perceptual understanding can ease the frustration during this period of difficult learning (Dolan, Epilogue).

The Dreyfus model (1980) suggests a new way of understanding the tension between theory and practice and offers avenues for making the most of that tension that is usually identified as the tension between school and work. Beginners must operate on abstract principles, formal models, and theories to get into the situation in a way that they can learn safely and efficiently. In contrast, experiential learning is posing and testing questions in real situations that deviate from expectations based upon theory and principles. Experience enables the expert to make rapid decisions based upon concrete examples. In addition to the use of past concrete examples as paradigms, the expert develops many perceptual distinctions that are not possible to learn or grasp conceptually. Thus, the theoretician must always depend on the practitioner for clinical knowledge development and for finding puzzles and questions that current theorizing does not predict or cover.

Early in the AMICAE Project, surveys of the ideal and real performance expectations of nurse educators, newly graduated nurses, and nursing service personnel (including experienced nurse clinicians), revealed little consensus or shared understanding among these three groups as to what the new nurse can and cannot do or should and should not be able to do. This lack of consensus is undoubtedly the source of much of the conflict and misunderstanding that currently exists among the three groups. Nursing service staff development programs may be geared to teach what new nurses believe they have already mastered. Nursing educators may be unduly pessimistic about the level of proficiency of their recent graduates. And beginning nurses may be bewildered and surprised at the low expectations that nursing service persons hold for them. One might assume that it would be hard for new nurses to succeed in an expectations climate which is so disparate from their own appraisal of their performance abilities.

Is the discrepancy between beginner nurse, nursing education, and nursing service performance expectations a crisis in confidence rather than in ability? This question was addressed, in part, by the 1979 AMICAE Project Self and Other Follow-Through Evaluation Study. In this study the newly graduated nurse was asked to complete a self-reported performance assessment and to select a nursing service colleague to fill out the same performance assessment tool. The performance items were the same as those in an earlier (1978) survey, but this time respondents were asked only for their *actual* appraisals, not their *ideal* expectations. It was predicted that the nursing service person's appraisal would be higher when the assessment referred to a particular new nurse rather than new nurses in general. This was, in fact, the case, as presented briefly below:

> At least 70 percent of the nursing service respondents rated their new graduates at the high proficiency level on 17 of the 80 skills. This is considerably higher than the appraisal made by nursing service respondents to the 1978

general survey that most new graduates do not perform *any* of the 80 skills at the high proficiency...The new graduates, when considering only their actual performance ability, and not their ideal standard, raised their assessment of their actual performance. At least 70 percent of the new graduates thought they performed at the high proficiency level on 24 of the 80 skills, as opposed to the 1978 general survey where new graduates thought they performed proficiently on only 15 of the skills. (Benner, et al., 1981, p. 18)

In effect, the newly graduated nurses rated their performance capabilities higher when considering only their actual level of proficiency, and the nursing service respondents raised their rating of these nurses' performance capability when considering only one particular nurse, and when they, too, considered only actual performance. These results would lend credence to the hypothesis that new nurses are stereotyped by nursing service personnel as being less competent than they actually are.*

Two explanations for the difference in new graduate performance appraisals and expectations by nursing service persons and nurse educators have been presented:

1. Negative stereotyping of the new graduate by nursing service persons; and

2. A basic difference between nursing service and nursing education in perception and understanding of skilled performance.

---

*These results have to be interpreted with caution since the return rate for the Self-and-Other reported assessment was only 18 percent compared to 46 percent and 52 percent return for new graduates and nursing service, respectively, for the 1978 general assessment.

The negative stereotyping or blanket appraisal of beginning nurses is based on the normal tendency to give blanket or global appraisals, so that if new nurses are found lacking in one area, they are considered deficient in all other areas. Nursing managers seem to be especially inclined toward this kind of generalization, since their appraisals of the new nurse are lower than the appraisals of the staff nurses who work more closely with the beginners. These findings suggest that nurse managers might do well to adjust and balance their negative appraisals in order to create a climate of success. The manager's perception may be distorted by exposure only to problems, with little opportunities to observe success, so the manager may need to deliberately seek out positive examples to balance the picture. It is easier to succeed in a climate where acceptance and expectations of success are the rule rather than the exception.

The second explanation for the disparity in nursing education and nursing service expectations is that the frame of reference for appraising the level of proficiency may be quite different for newly graduated nurses, nurse educators, and nursing service personnel. New nurses and nurse educators may judge proficiency within a "return demonstration" in a skills lab context, whereas the nursing service person is apt to judge proficiency with a range of patient complexity and variability in mind. It was this second explanation that led to the systematic comparison of differences between expert and novice clinicians' perceptions and descriptions of clinical situations and to examination of what the nurse clinician learns from experience. But, first, to understand the differences between the educator's and service person's views of skill acquisition, it is useful to look at the disparities between formal and informal views of the organization.

Schein's (1968) work on organization socialization is a key resource for most studies of professional and occupational socialization. Schein, like other educators, tends to emphasize formal, conceptual knowledge. He draws a sharp contrast between the values of the professional business school and the organizational realities. He sees errors in the "ad hoc wisdom" proffered in the organization that the business school faculty has taught the business student to avoid. He sees virtue in the pure rationality and emotional neutrality taught in the business school and fears that, upon going to work, the graduate will be oversocialized so that these virtues are lost. He argues for creative individualism in which the occupational entrant adopts only pivotal values within the organization and eschews the peripheral values. Schein's position as an educator of professional managers mirrors the position of other educators of professionals, including nurses.

In the abstract, Schein's advice sounds plausible, but in reality it is difficult to follow since organizations operate more like cultures than rationalized organization charts. Few of the core values are explicit in the professional school *or* in the work organization. Socialization works because there is a taken-for-granted background of assumptions and values that one cannot get completely clear about or make completely explicit. Therefore, one cannot clearly choose which values will be pursued and which will be rejected. Situational adjustment will cause one to take up many practices that embody values one does not recognize or freely choose.

The norms and policies of complex social organizations can never be totally clear or explicit; they remain broad and functionally vague. Thus, despite efforts at value clarification and rationalization to make institutional objectives explicit, many subtle expectations will remain unnamed (Benner & Benner, 1979). As Breed (1955) points out in his analysis of a newsroom, this ambiguity provides the flexibility necessary in organizational settings:

> The norms of policy are not always entirely clear, just as many norms are vague and unstructured. Policy is covert and by nature has large scope. . . . Policy, if worked out explicitly, would have to include motivations, reasons, alternatives, historical developments, and other complicating material. Thus, a twilight zone permitting a range of deviation appears. (p. 333)

While organizational activity presses toward increased clarity and increased rationalization, at least two things would happen (Benner & Benner, 1979) if it were possible to remove all ambiguity and implicit expectations from organizational life:

1. The system would lose its interpretive power and flexibility. It would resemble the limited problem-solving capability of the computer, which requires explicitly stated rules for all operations.* Patient care exists in complex environments. It is never context-free or static. Broad, vaguely outlined policy allows for the greatest interpretation and adaptation to changing complex contingencies.

2. There is not enough space and time to make all of the expectations generated in organizational contexts explicit. To do that would require all of the available

---

*For further description and analysis of the limits of formalization see: Dreyfus, Hubert, *What Computers Can't Do: The Limits of Artificial Intelligence*, New York: Harper and Row, 1972.

organizational space and time for list making and rule generation.

It is useful to make rules explicit so that procedures can be coordinated and carried out with some degree of quality control. Indeed, a major strategy for reducing conflict in organizations is to formalize rules and to write out policies. But there is a limit to what can and should be made explicit, as exemplified by the nurse who would follow the written nursing care plan to the letter without assessing changes in the patient or environment that may have occurred since the plan was written. Such a nurse would have lost the ability to grasp distinctions and exceptions without precise written policy and would be considered unsafe to practice.

As we have pointed out earlier, the novice operates on abstract principles and formal models and theories (Dreyfus & Dreyfus, 1980; Dreyfus, 1981). These serve as powerful tools for the beginner to get into the situation so that learning can be achieved efficiently. For example, the beginning pilot is initially taught all the operational procedures in the form of rules; as his or her skills progress, the rules can be elaborated upon by guidelines; and finally, as proficiency is achieved, maxims can be used. The expert uses concrete examples much as the scientist uses paradigms to guide research. These exemplars (concrete examples) are much richer than any formal model could capture, since perceptual distinctions are grasped as well as conceptual issues. This level of performance is based on the maximum grasp of the situation and can occur only with concrete experience (Dreyfus & Dreyfus, 1980).

There has been a devaluing and ignoring of the knowledge embodied in the skilled performance of the expert nurse clinician. Yet if that knowledge is taken seriously, then the understanding of "reality shock" changes. Reality shock is redefined as that uncomfortable process of gaining experiential learning that cannot be conveyed by formal models, formal theories, or forecasts about what a situation will be like. Adlai Stevenson once described experience this way:

> A knowledge not gained by words but by touch, sight, sound, victories, failures, sleeplessness, devotions, love — the human experiences and emotions of this earth and of oneself and other men.

It is evident that professional socialization in nursing and in medicine is undergoing change. In the past, nurse educators in their quest for professionalization have, like Schein, preferred rationalized, formal decision-making models. Thus, training in decision making in nursing education became decontextualized; the exigencies and constraints of the workplace were omitted. Efforts are now underway to change this practice and enrich educational programs with more realistic practice in decision making (Kramer, 1974; Limon, Spencer, & Waters, 1981).

13 | The Quest for a New Identity and New Entitlement in Nursing

Work attitudes and relationships are changing. Individuals are demanding more from their work situation. The meaning of success is changing so that the individual who sacrifices a high quality of lifestyle, friendships, and health for economic security and status is no longer considered unquestionably successful. There are more dual-career families, and new negotiations between the sexes are carried out. Yankelovich (1974) has called this the era of entitlement, the growth of a broad new agenda of "social rights." Much of the change might sound like narcissism if the worker did not include meaningful work in the sense of psychological fulfillment, not just pleasure seeking. Workers want to feel proud of their work; they want to feel competent.

Yankelovich (1974) outlines three psychological benefits people would like to gain from their work:

1. The opportunity to advance to more interesting, varied, and more satisfying work that also pays better and wins more recognition than the current job.

2. The desire to do a good job at whatever one is doing.
3. The yearning to find self-fulfillment through "meaningful work." By meaningful work people usually mean:
   (a) work in which they can become involved, committed, and interested;
   (b) work that challenges them to the utmost of their capabilities; and
   (c) participation in decision making. (p. 35)

Nursing can offer ways to meet all of these psychological requirements. However, nurses are not adequately recognized — by consumers, physicians, administrators, and sometimes even their own colleagues — for the highly responsible, difficult, and significant work they do. This is a lag in recognition of their worth rather than a lack of responsible, significant roles. Nurses make life-and-death decisions and possess an increasingly specialized body of knowledge.

That nurses desire to do a good job is evident in the following quote from a nursing dropout (Godfrey, 1975):

> To keep my sanity and marriage, I left nursing. The chronic understaffing, frequent shift changes, and weekend work exhausted me and created tension with my wife. When I had to ask my doctor for Valium so I could face going to work, I decided it was time to get out.
>
> I now earn twice my nursing salary, but I still think of going back. The emotional rewards in nursing are worth more than my present higher salary, *but only if I am allowed time to meet my patients' needs.* (p. 90)

This nurse's comments illustrate the psychology of entitlement well. They point to the potential in nursing for increased job satisfaction and decreased turnover, once there is more adequate staffing and increased stability. These comments also point up the fact that nurses' motivation to do a good job is heightened by the serious, life-threatening consequences of not doing a good job.

According to the Yankelovich criteria, nursing provides meaningful work, work in which one can become involved, and work that challenges one's capabilities. But the nurse's efficacy is blocked by a lack of shared decision making. Within the hospital social system nurses are usually excluded from governing boards and decision-making committees, and they are not recognized for their own clinical decision making. But this tradition can be changed so that nurses will be recognized for their input as members of the governing boards, committees, and clinical decision-making teams. The national hearings by the National Commission on Nursing attest to nurses' need to be included in collaborative decision making within the hospital system (Flanagan, 1981).

Advanced scientific knowledge and technology have changed both illness and health care and, as a physician and medical school professor testified at the hearing of the National Commission on Nursing, the nursing role has been enlarged:

> One major adaptation to this explosive change has been the steadily progressive shifting of responsibility and actual work from the doctor to the nurse, sometimes in a planned orderly fashion but more often in staccato, unplanned crescendo, unappreciated and uncompensated in resource allocation. The intern and the nurse simply do more, are constantly being stretched further because today's adjustments require statistical proof of yesterday's unmet needs to compete for tomorrow's shrinking dollars. (Flanagan, 1981, p. 12)

The impact of the lack of recognition of nursing's expanded responsibilities is felt keenly by the new recruit to the profession. The beginning nurses who participated in this study grappled with their personal and societal image and tried to reconcile that image with their actual work demands and accomplishments. One recently graduated nurse's statement is typical:

> One of the hardest things I am dealing with is the fact that I'm a nurse. My friends don't understand why I choose nursing and they think that what I do is demeaning. I get exasperated and explain that I deal with important life-and-death issues daily and that I get a great deal of satisfaction in the kinds of human contact and relationships that I have in my work. I don't know when I will personally feel OK about being a nurse or, as my friends say, "just being a nurse," but I haven't arrived yet.

This presents society, nurses, physicians, and hospital administrators with a charge to re-evaluate the functions and importance of nursing. Until nursing is recognized and rewarded for its contributions by all sectors, nurses will continue to grapple with their sense of self-worth, identity, and commitment. Increased careerism and career opportunities for women make the status inequities, lack of shared governance, and career deprivations of hospital nursing stand out for both the new recruit and the experienced nurse, even though they may find the practice of nursing personally satisfying and rewarding.

The extensive documentation of actual nursing practice in today's acute care hospital that has been presented in this book illustrates the complex, central role nurses play in the patient's recovery. The exemplars illustrate the expanded responsibility of the nurse. The formal models used by educators and the policy and "standards of care" language often used by nurse managers overlook much of what nurses actually do; they ignore nurses' discretionary judgment and clinical expertise. At best, the competent level of nursing practice is the one captured in written standards and guidelines. Until nurses' language and their documentation of nursing functions match the reality of nursing practice, the recognition lag in nursing will continue within nursing itself.

Meaningful Incentives and Reward Systems

Restructuring and sweeping changes are called for if clinical nursing as a career is to be brought in step with career opportunities in other fields. Nursing faces the risk of brain drain as the most talented potential nurses select other fields that offer not only higher salaries but also opportunities for career development and a share in policy decisions. Entitlement, recognition, and rewards commensurate with knowledge, skill, and responsibility, however, *are* possible in nursing.

The following incentives and rewards are identified as crucial to restructuring hospital nursing practice:

1. Retention and career development for beginning and midcareer nurses in positions that have clinical input.
2. A clinical promotion system that integrates clinical knowledge development and clinical career development.
3. Increased collaborative relationships between physicians and nurses.
4. Increased recognition of the significance of the nursing role in patient care.

Most hospitals have allocated only relatively small amounts of money to research and development in nursing care and, when funds are limited, resources for staff development are often the first to be cut. Furthermore, these limited resources have been spent on orienting new employees and managing high turnover. Little attention has been given to the development of the midcareer nurse clinician who is a key figure in the provision of expert nursing care and the development of clinical knowledge. This lack of attention to clinical knowledge development and career development for the midcareer employee is a major barrier to the retention of expert nurse clinicians at the patient's bedside (Benner & Wrubel, 1982).

From the Dreyfus model it is predicted that the nurse who has reached the competent level of skill acquisition is best taught by demonstration and case studies offered by the proficient or expert level practitioner. Thus, the first requirement for clinical knowledge development is the retention and continued development of the experienced nurse clinician. Provision for exchange about clinical experiences across levels of education and experience can promote this development.

Research into and validation of nursing practice can be conducted most fruitfully in situations where a well-articulated background of practices and assumptions exists that can be systematically tested. Nurses themselves have not valued their observational powers and clinical experience sufficiently to engage in a systematic program of documenting what they learn from their practice. The applications that will be presented in the epilogue illustrate that such clinical documentation can be integrated into nursing practice.

As part of their quest of entitlement, nurses want to do a good job. The complexity of the patient assessments and interventions illustrated in Chapter 3 calls for ways to enrich and refine experiential learning. Both knowledge utilization (introduction into practice of the latest advances in research and technology) and clinical knowledge development (the description and systematic study of experiential learning) must be addressed by nursing departments (Benner & Wrubel, 1982). Indeed, the education and development function of hospitals must expand to meet the increased knowledge utilization and development needs of the nursing department.

Much attention is given in hospitals and in the literature to the school-to-work transition of newly graduated nurses. As illustrated in the description of the advanced beginner's level of skill acquisition, attention must be given to the acquisition of refined clinical judgment by enabling comparison of the advanced beginner's judgments with those of the experienced clinician; this is how a sense of salience is gained. Time and multiple examples are required. But it is also crucial that the new nurse be presented with a challenging first job—one that stretches his or her abilities (Benner & Benner, 1979).

Research in other fields indicates that one of the most successful retention strategies for the new recruit is a challenging first job. Hall and Hall (1976) and Berlew and Hall (1966) found that the more challenging a person's job during the first year, the more successful that person will be five or seven years later. Bray, Campbell, and Grant (1974), in a study of managers, also found that one of the strongest predictors of later career success is a challenging, stimulating first job. Thus caution is needed in providing support for clinical knowledge development for beginning nurses. They should not be so protected that they are prevented from experiencing challenge and success sufficient to gain a sense of commitment and identity with the organization.

A Clinical Promotion System

Many nursing service departments are now experimenting with clinical promotion opportunities in order to convert direct patient care positions into attractive, long-term career options (Bracken & Chestmann, 1978; Mintel & Rhodes, 1977; Colavecchio, Tescher, & Scalzi, 1974). To be effective, these clinical promotions must be based on increased levels of skill acquisition and knowledge. Walton (1975) outlines the following guidelines for career development, noting that attention needs to be given to:

1. The extent to which the worker's assignment contributes to maintaining and expanding his/her capabilities rather than leading to obsolescence.
2. The degree to which expanded on, newly acquired knowledge and skill can be utilized in future work assignments.
3. The availability of opportunities to advance in the organization on career terms which peers, family members, or associates recognize. (p. 32)

As noted earlier, many of the current management practices and written policies in nursing departments have been designed to decrease the impact of chronically high staff turnover; written policies and procedures, for example, are developed to limit the dangers inherent in giving inexperienced nurses discretionary powers beyond their knowledge and experience levels. But these same safety-oriented policies and procedures can frustrate the expert nurse clinician who uses much more discretionary judgment. Formal recognition of the increased discretionary judgment and responsibility of the expert nurse would sanction and reward this advanced level of performance.

For clinical promotions to have meaning for the individual and the organization, they must be based upon demonstrated clinical knowledge and performance. Patient outcomes and patient appraisals as well as nurse and physician colleague appraisals will have to be gathered to adequately document and reward excellence. Nurses themselves can also be encouraged to document and reward the excellence illustrated in the Epilogue. Such documentation could be done in promotion portfolios.

Salary structures must reflect the advancement indicated by the clinical promotion ladder. The salary increments must be comparable to administrative promotions and allow for increments over a period of 20 years. Currently, a serious wage compression exists in positions of direct patient care. In an era with cost containment pressures, a change in salary structure entails reallocation of funds and better personnel resource management.

Clinical promotions, to be real promotions and not just wage increases, must offer new challenge and variety to the nurse's role; creative experimentation is called for. Attention might be given to increasing the nurse's clinical teaching functions on the patient care unit, or enabling her or him to share in such matters as consultation; trouble-shooting specific, recurring clinical problems; and hospitalwide committee work as possible options for promoting a sense of challenge and empowerment. Finally, as mentioned earlier, formal acknowledgement of increased discretionary judgment should accompany the clinical promotion.

Increased Collaborative Relationships

Nursing has been doing much these past years to increase the relative status of nurses vis-a-vis physicians. The experience of nurses in their work is highly affected by their relationships with physicians. Both physicians and nurses must work on developing more collaborative relationships in their educational programs and in the work settings.

Nursing administration and hospital administration must provide leadership and policies that will foster such collaboration. Nurses must have efficient, responsive channels for reporting medically urgent patient problems. Nurses who fail to obtain a timely or appropriate response from the physician in charge and who find existing communication channels ponderous or laden with strong negative social sanctions find their position untenable and their effectiveness limited. In life-and-death matters, responsibility cannot be constrained within formal lines of authority. The nurse who reports an urgent need without getting an effective response is left with feelings of guilt, moral outrage, and helplessness.

Increased Recognition

The lack of societal and professional recognition of the significance of the nursing role for patient recovery must be combatted on many fronts. It is crucial that descriptions of nursing practice match the significance and scope of nursing as it is practiced in the hospital setting. Diers (1980) calls attention to this problem when she says:

> Nursing cannot be explained by conceptual jargon . . . .
> If we are confused, it may be because we are swayed by the

demands of academe for pomposity; of management for simple explanations and rules; of professional colleagues for obsequiousness; of a sexist society for conformity.

The actual performance of the expert nurse clinician outstrips most descriptions of nursing practice found in formal models. Nurses must change the way they describe what they do in actual practice.

14 | Excellence and Power in Clinical Nursing Practice

    I have left the exemplars in the same "spoken" language as they were delivered, because I did not want to inadvertently strip away the evidence of concern and advocacy for the patient expressed in the telling of these stories. Nurses were coached to include intentions and to avoid using the usual cryptic reporting language that is used to save time. These exemplars illustrate excellence and power in nursing. Excellence requires commitment and involvement, but it also requires power. Since caring is central to nursing, then power without excellence is an anathema.

    I am concerned when I hear nurses say that the very qualities essential to their caring role are the source of their powerlessness in the male-dominated hospital hierarchy. Such a statement disparages feminine qualities and elevates a masculine view of power, one that emphasizes competitiveness, domination, and control. But to define *power* or *nursing* exclusively in traditional masculine or feminine terms is a mistake. The disparagement of feminine perspectives on power is based upon the misguided assumption that feminine values have kept women and nursing subservient, rather than recognizing that society's devaluing of and discrimination against women are the sources of the problem. The former view — the misguided assumption — blames the victim and promises that discrimination will stop when women abandon what they value and learn to play the power games like men do. It mistakes observations of a descriptive sociology for an explanation of the way things are.

To adopt a definition of power that excludes the power of caring does not gain the power of self-determination. Adopting coercive, dominating notions of power or strictly public-relations approaches abandons the values and commitments required for powerful caring and excellence; it adopts the pathologies inherent in a unipolar view. Gilligan (1982, 1983) points out that the ethics of care and responsibility differ from the ethics of rights and justice (see also Sandel, 1982). Greer (1973) has also voiced this concern:

> If women understand by emancipation the adoption of the masculine role, then we are lost indeed. If women can supply no counterbalance to the blindness of male drive, the aggressive society will run to its lunatic extremes at ever-escalating speed. Who will safeguard the despised animal faculties of compassion, empathy, innocence, and sensuality? (pp. 411–12)

Nursing is facing profound changes in self-interpretation. In the past, service was connected to subservience, and self-sacrifice was linked to self-effacement. Everyone will gain if the notions of self-effacement and unnecessary self-sacrifice are dropped. (I say unnecessary self-sacrifice, because the demands of nursing are large ones. The pain, risks, and dangers encountered are sometimes great and cannot be experienced without personal cost.)

The nurses who took part in this study have offered us glimpses of the nature of the power that resides in caring. They have used their power to empower their patients—not to dominate, coerce, or control them. But this relationship is highly contextual. To empower, nurses sometimes border on coercion as they coach and prompt the patient to engage in painful tasks that patients would not readily undertake on their own. The difference between empowerment and domination can be understood only if the nurse–patient relationship and the situation are understood. Caring out of context will always be controversial, because caring is local, specific, and individual.

The nurses in this study found safety in their use of power by genuinely caring for their patients. They identified with their patients by imagining themselves or their family members in the same predicament, and they reminded themselves of the "otherness" of the patient when such identification distorted their caring. There was a notable absence of smugness about their caring. They did not know if their care would always be available, nor did they assume that they would always know how to offer the most caring responses.

I concluded that this lack of smugness is a mark of the wisdom and humility that comes with experience. Nurses often deal with dilemmas rather than with easily solved "problems." Sometimes their risk-taking in the context of genuine concern shocked them, and it was unclear to both the nurses and the researchers what made the risky intervention work. One thing *is* clear: Almost no intervention will work if the nurse–patient relationship is not based on mutual respect and genuine caring.

I have identified six different qualities of power associated with the caring provided by the nurses participating in this study: transformative, integrative, advocacy, healing, participative/affirmative, and problem solving.

❘ Transformative Power

The transformative power of caring was well illustrated by the exemplar describing the man who was tired of people "doing" things to him. He was depressed and the nurse who was also a friend gave him a stern lecture, declaring that he did have the power to choose how he would respond to his circumstance; that he had indeed already exercised that power by taking his care into his own hands and seeking a transfer to the medical center. This somewhat risky "lecture" from a position of mutual trust and a caring attitude was enough to transform the patient's sense of possibility. In effect, it transformed his world into one that he could once again participate in. It was evident that his world had been transformed the next day as he sat in the hall, laughing and smiling, and told the nurse: "You were right! I'm just going to choose to be here and let all of you help me get well as fast as I can!"

A second example of the transformative or world-changing power was described in a clinical knowledge development seminar. A young man had returned to thank the nurses who had cared for him during a protracted complicated illness; their genuine and imaginative care during his long period of pain and helplessness had made a profound impression on him. He wanted to tell them that their care had changed his world. He had never imagined that anyone could have been as helpless, unattractive, and with so little to offer in the way of social exchange as he had been, and yet be so cared for. He had a new, perceptually grounded faith in his fellow human beings. His former perspective that life is a contract and you get only what you earn had broadened to a view that sometimes you get what you are not able to ask or barter for. He never wanted to go back to that extremely helpless state, but the care he received during that period permanently changed his understanding of caring.

Integrative Caring

Caring can also reintegrate the individual into his or her own social world. In patient care situations where a prolonged or permanent disability is inevitable, the nurse is often instrumental in helping patients maximize their ability to continue with meaningful life activities despite their limitations. This was the case with the nurse who helped the woman who was confined to her bedroom after a stroke. The nurse helped the woman rejoin her family, even though it was considered risky at the time. The integrative power of caring was also evident in the exemplar describing the nurse who, with the help of the Muscular Dystrophy Association, helped a high school student return to school and to his job as a sports announcer.

In both exemplars, the nurses were instrumental in assessing the importance of helping the patient to continue with normal activity to minimize the isolation, loss of meaning, and inactivity. In both cases, the choices contained risk, and the risks were explored. But the nurses offered the option of reintegration by providing the patients and families with new possibilities in the midst of deprivation and loss.

211

| Advocacy

Patients and families frequently need the nurse to run
defense for them. They may be mystified by the medical
jargon, or their understanding may be blocked by fear.
The nurse can interpret patient to doctor and doctor to
patient. I call this kind of power *advocacy power*. It is
the kind of power that removes obstacles or stands
alongside and enables. Enabling, advocacy power was
illustrated by the nurse who convinced the physician
that he should delay giving medications that would
take away a patient's own respiratory drive, even
though his hyperventilation was a serious problem and
his blood gases were compromised. The nurse helped
the young man to calm down and thus maintain control
over his one last set of functioning muscles. The nurse's
own words depict this kind of powerful caring best and
bear repeating here:

It took three and a half hours before he began to relax. He needed
to understand what had happened, and was presently happening
to him. He needed to be reassured, and most of all to learn to
trust us. He needed to know what the future might hold for him.
He needed to know that we cared about *him*, as an individual,
not just another helpless patient. As he began to comprehend
these things, he learned to trust us. That was the key. He needed
to be involved, not just prescribed to. He felt so very
helpless . . . . The point was made by one simple statement he
mouthed to me late in the day . . . when he had a respiratory rate
in the 20s, and he was no longer threatened with having the few
remaining functional muscles chemically paralyzed: His words
were: "Thank you. You've really helped me a lot. I don't want to
imagine what would have happened to me if you weren't here
and hadn't cared."

212

Healing Power

The above example also illustrates the healing power of caring. Nurses establish a healing relationship and create a healing climate by: (1) mobilizing hope in themselves, the staff, and the patient; (2) finding an interpretation or understanding of the situation (e.g., illness, pain, fear, or other stressful emotion) that is acceptable and clarifying to the patient; and (3) assisting the patient to use social, emotional, and spiritual support. The healing power of the nurse–patient relationship was also illustrated in the exemplar about the young woman caught in conflict and confusion about choosing a therapy.

A healing relationship solicits the patient's internal and external resources and empowers the patient by bringing hope, confidence, and trust. The study of endorphins and Norman Cousins' (1976, 1983) description of his recovery have brought new attention to the personal and social side of recovery and given new respectability to the "placebo effect." It is unclear how often technological causes have been given undue credit in recovery, while the real cause was much more interactive with a healing relationship.

Participative/Affirmative Power

It may sound as though these powerful ways of caring will lead to only one thing: that dreaded modern disease called burnout. The notion of burnout is based on the naive metaphor of élan vital—the notion that a person has only so much life force, only so much of the precious juices of caring. Selye (1969) uses the analogy of the bank account; this is only a modern variation on the élan vital theme.

Although it is true that caretakers must take care of themselves, must have respites, vacations, fun, reasonable workloads, and equitable salaries, it is *not* true that the best protection against burnout lies in distancing and control strategies—that is, protection against caring. I don't think these are effective strategies because they only weakly shield the caregiver from the pain, take a tremendous amount of energy, and prevent appropriation of the resources available in the situation. The exemplar describing the nurse who provides comfort and presences herself with family during the wife–mother's last moments of life illustrates the best antidote to burnout in the work setting; engagement and involvement that enable the nurse to draw on the resources in the demanding situation. I call this the participative/affirmative power of caring.

In participating, this nurse was able to use the meanings and resources inherent in this poignant event. In caring, she not only experienced pain, but also strength and affirmation. She learned first-hand about a human possibility that many never experience or witness and she felt affirmed and stronger for it. One could imagine that a detached, avoiding approach would have offered only frail protection and no positive resources such as the participative and affirmative power of caring that this nurse gained.

Problem Solving

Finally, a caring, involved stance is the prerequisite for expert, creative problem solving. This is because the most difficult problems to solve require perceptual ability as well as conceptual reasoning, and perception requires engagement and attentiveness. People who are especially ego-involved have an uncanny ability to hear their name at a distance in a crowded room. Similarly, a committed stance provides a sensitivity to cues that allows persons to search for solutions and even makes it possible to recognize a solution when they are not directly looking for it. Polanyi (1958) has persuasively described the role of intellectual passion and the tacit dimension for expert human problem solving. Perceptual awareness precedes conceptual awareness. For example, nurses become experts in reading patients' faces and in discerning global, subtle changes before they are documentable by explicit vital signs such as changes in EKG or blood pressure.

Expertise depends on a meaningful engagement in the situation. The expert rapidly grasps the problem by seeing it in relation to past similar and dissimilar situations and rapidly hones in on the correct region of the problem. The beginner, in contrast, must rely on detached, deliberate considerations of as many variables as possible. The best example of this is the contrast between the medical student and the consulting specialist. The medical student takes an elaborate history and physical that takes into account every possible contributing factor, while the specialist who asks only a few questions zeroes in on the accurate region of the problem.

A preference for detached, reflective reasoning and formal, explicit knowledge overlooks the role of caring with its attendant emotions — vague feelings, hunches, a sense that something is not right — or the creative search and cue sensitivity that occur as a result of caring. The power of caring is underestimated and undervalued in this era when status, mastery, control, and knowledge (interpreted as detached, reflective thinking) are seen as the sources of power. But such a view of power is unipolar and not the most adaptive one. To abandon the power inherent in caring relationships is to sell out but, worse yet, it is to become alienated from our own identity and to thwart our own excellence. Ultimately, our power in terms of mastery, status, and control over our own practice depends upon excellence.

Nursing without caring is powerful and devastating. Nurses can have enormous power over how a patient will spend the first or last hours on earth. Although nurses have done much to ensure that the first moments of life are spent with loving parents, the last hours are all too often spent in restraints or resisting a retention catheter that has been put in place for the health care personnel's convenience. Perhaps the most indicting example of abused power was portrayed in the book (Kesey, 1962) and movie, *One Flew Over the Cuckoo's Nest*.

Nurses do have power, though they exert their power from a position of low status in the hierarchy. They are the ones who are there, and they know how to work the system. A patient can have a very skilled, knowledgeable physician, but if the nurse is lacking in diagnostic, monitoring, or therapeutic skills — and, most serious of all, if the nurse does not care — the patient's chances for recovery, or for dignity and comfort in dying, are slim. It is important to clarify this negative side of the nurse's power because, like the positive side, it is a corrective for society's lag in recognizing the importance of nursing to healing.

Nursing offers crucial services that require high intelligence, a thorough and sound educational base, and firm grounding in the ethics of both rights and justice and care and responsibility (Gilligan, 1982; 1983; Sandel, 1982).

Structural or linear process descriptions or any context-stripping approach runs the risk of overlooking or mistaking the quality of caring. Steinbeck (1941) has vividly captured the mistakes inherent in decontextualized objectivity:

> The Mexican Sierra has 17 plus 9 spines in the dorsal fin. These can easily be counted, but if the sierra strikes hard on the line so that our hands are burned, if the fish sounds and nearly escapes and finally comes in over the rail, his colors pulsing and his tail beating in the air, a whole new relational externality has come into being — an entity which is more than the sum of the fish plus the fisherman. The only way to count the spines of the sierra unaffected by this second relational reality is to sit in a laboratory, open an evil-smelling jar, remove a stiff colorless fish from the formalin solution, count the spines and write the truth. . . There you have recorded a reality that cannot be assailed — probably the least important reality concerning the fish or yourself. . .It is good to know what you are doing. The man with this pickled fish has set down one truth and recorded in his experience many lies. The fish is not that color, that texture, that dead, nor does he smell that way.

The accounts in this book have been presented as an attempt to look at the whole, to include the content, action, and context. This research explores the meanings embedded in nursing practice; it is an attempt to make practice *primary*. To do this, two assumptions of naturalism were abandoned (Taylor, 1982):

1. that meaning can be seen in terms of representation of an independent reality (based on the 17th-century philosophers, Hobbes and Locke). Such a view inevitably treats the research subject as an object and ignores our everyday access to our world through

217

skill, through direct perceptual grasp, and through the knowing that comes from an involved, committed human relationship.

2. that theory can be generated from the standpoint of a monological observer, who stands outside the situation and has private meanings that are then tested or matched with public activities.

This position ignores the fact that the researcher is a self-interpreting human being who participates in a shared background of common meanings that can be made public through dialogue (Heidegger, 1962; Palmer, 1969). In this latter view, even basic needs are imbued with meaning and not really separable from them.

The research reported in this book has taken a dialogical stance, and the point of the inquiry has been to uncover meanings and knowledge embedded in skilled practice. By bringing these meanings, skills, and knowledge into public discourse, new knowledge and understanding are constituted, as Taylor (1982) points out:

> Language doesn't only serve to describe or represent things. Rather there are some phenomena, central to human life, which are partly constituted by language . . . The public space between us is founded on and shaped by our language; the fact that there is such a thing is due to our being language animals. And our typically human concerns only exist through articulation and expression. . . . It does not follow [from this] that our feelings can be shaped at will by the descriptions that we offer. Feelings are rather shaped by the descriptions that seem to us adequate. . . . The formulations we offer of our concerns are put forward in an attempt to get it right. . . That is, we recognize that self-descriptions can be more or less clairvoyant, or deluded or blind, or deep, or shallow, and so

on. . . .But it is not only our feelings which are partly constituted by our self-descriptions. So are our relations, the kinds of footings we can be on with each other. (pp. 305–6)

Put simply, we both shape and are shaped by our language. Our public language about nursing has grown too constricted and sterile as a result of monological theories and an attempt to develop a general, context-free language to cover the local and individual contingencies in nursing. The emphasis on structure and process has caused us to ignore the context, the content, and functions of nursing. This is dangerous because it puts us on a new footing with our patients and with ourselves. It puts us in the precarious position of trivializing the distress of our patients, of turning dilemmas and distress into "problems" to be solved (Lazarus, in press). It is encouraging to find that expert practice is wiser than our formulations and formal models. These nurses took the distress of their patients seriously.

Our language needs to be enriched by a new immersion in the actual practice of nursing. The linear ideal that theory must be generated first and then applied to nursing has given us a deficit view of nursing practice, allowing us to see only the gaps. We cannot afford to ignore knowledge gained from clinical experience by viewing it only from simplified models or from idealized, decontextualized views of practice. Nor can we afford to attend to and legitimize only what we learn from scientific experiments; the scope and complexity of our practice are too extensive for this. We have to choose our experiments wisely so that they enlighten our controversies and questions arising from our experience. For the sake of economy, we need to avoid documenting the obvious and agreed-upon issues and focus our search on the confusing and conflicting ones.

Carefully selected research programs, however, depend on clinicians being conversant with one another about what they are learning from their clinical experience. Knowledge utilization has been emphasized at the expense of the clinical knowledge development. If we are to humanize care in the midst of highly technical medicine, we must master the technology. We must also critique the technology and not view it as the ultimate resource in recovery, dignity, and health. As an antidote to a purely technical view of health and power, we must understand and unleash the power of caring, the power of excellence.

Epilogue:
Practical Applications

      In the preface, I stated that this work has been a dialogue with nurses and nursing; this chapter represents a part of the dialogue. This work has grown, as nurses in education and service have applied it in their various settings. I can think of no better way to present practical applications than to have the people who have made the applications present their own work. In each case these authors have had advanced previews of this work in the form of first drafts of manuscripts, workshops, and/or direct participation in the AMICAE project. They have not, however, had the advantage of talking to one another so that they could compare their experiences. Their articles reflect diversities and local innovations. Their first-hand reports offer ideas and advice on implementing and refining the ideas presented in this book.

      Deborah Gordon's article is an example of a particular research study that was based on this work. Dr. Gordon is a medical anthropologist who was a research associate on the AMICAE project and extended the lines of inquiry pursued in the project to her own research for her doctoral dissertation. Gordon examines the practices of formalization in an urban medical center setting. She analyzes the functions and dangers of specific formal models as they are used on two medical-surgical nursing units. Her provocative analysis challenges nurses to take control of their formal models as tools to be mastered instead of the tools themselves becoming the masters.

Ann Huntsman and her colleagues in staff development at El Camino Hospital, Mountain View, California, describe their efforts to establish a ladder for clinical promotion based upon the Dreyfus model of skill acquisition. This article presents an inside look at the development of a peer review process that focuses on the acutal practice of the nurse: as part of her evaluation profile for peer review, the nurse presents exemplars from her own practice that reflect excellence. The nurses at El Camino Hospital participated in the AMI-CAE project and as a result sought ways of incorporating interpretive evaluation strategies into their peer review process.

These nurses had the foresight to save the exemplars from the peer review profiles and, as they accumulate, the nurses will have an unusual opportunity for self-study. What is not easily documented at this point are the professional development benefits accrued by nurses taking the time to consider their own practice seriously as they examine it with their peers. Just as nursing slips into invisible spaces, the glue that holds the hospital together, these nurses initially presented "invisible" descriptions of their practice; they found it hard to take credit for their contributions to patient welfare and recovery. They hid behind cryptic analytic jargon and impersonal third person descriptions. With time the processes of presenting their own practice and taking credit for their contributions have become easier. The closing of the recognition lag has and must begin with nurses themselves. Only as we begin to acknowledge and better understand our role will we become more understandable to others. The high level of judgment and risk taking is now clearly being presented in the peer review process and is becoming more evident to nurses and administrators.

Jeanette Ullery, Director of Staff Development, St. Luke's Regional Medical Center, Boise, Idaho, presents an approach to clinical knowledge development seminars that began as a symposium. Facilitators have been trained for each nursing unit, and aspects of clinical knowledge are systematically explored in small groups as nurses present and compare exemplars from their current practice where they have learned something new or where they have made a difference in patient care. This strategy requires training for both the facilitators and participants. At first, events in practice are considered too "ordinary" or too specialized to be presented. But with time, nurses begin to discover common meanings and common experiences. Now that this program has been in effect for one year, time will be spent looking at commonalities and trends evident in particular patient populations. This group is ready to move from pure description to more synthesis and explanation.

Mary Fenton is an Associate Professor at the University of Texas Medical Branch at Galveston. She describes an innovative evaluative research study that used an interpretive methodology to describe and evaluate the performance of master's prepared clinical specialists. This evaluation strategy identifies areas of skilled performance and deficits as described and identified in small group interviews and participant observation. This project was conducted by the faculty themselves, so that the latter have new first-hand knowledge about the resources, demands, and constraints that the clinical specialists they prepare confront in their actual practice. As a side benefit, faculty members have gained new material for case studies drawn from recent practice episodes.

Finally, Kathy Dolan, Assistant Director of Nursing Education and Research, Nursing Service, at University of California San Francisco Medical Center describes practical applications of this work for the new graduate orientation program, for preceptor training, and for teaching the experienced nurse. Dolan's article points out that focusing on clinical practice can be a means of building bridges between nursing service and nursing education. Her article reflects her own level of participating in and extending this work and offers concrete examples that will be useful to administrators, staff development personnel, and to newly graduated nurses.

Research Application: Identifying the Use and Misuse of Formal Models in Nursing Practice

by Deborah R. Gordon, Ph.D.
Medical Anthropology Program
University of California, San Francisco

Research into clinical nursing practice is essential for critical evaluation of practice, for understanding what is optimal nursing care, and for learning how best to provide it. Research progresses through new concepts, theories, paradigms, and methods that in turn make new data visible. Such was the case in the research I conducted as an anthropologist with the AMICAE project, as developed and presented by Patricia Benner in this book. Using such concepts as formal models, experience, novice, and expert, a great deal of new data became visible, understandable, and open for critical review.

Employing anthropological methods of observation and interview, I studied two general surgical units over a two-year period — units characterized during the time of study by high rates of nursing turnover and consequently large proportions of newly graduated nurses.* The nursing staff was predominantly R.N., the model

---

*In the interest of maintaining anonymity, identifying characteristics of the research site have been changed.

of care was modified primary nursing, and the units were organized around 12-hour shifts. Clinical nursing was structured in the form of a ladder and consisted of Staff Nurse I, II, III, and IV positions. In observing these units, I was able to see how the transition from novice to expert was approached and encouraged, how expertise was defined and developed, and the obstacles to its development. I was also able to see how nursing turnover, so very frequent, had actually become part of the culture of these units: how the units were oriented toward nurses passing through; how interchangeability of nurses was esteemed and fostered; and how a structured passage from entry to departure had been formed (Gordon, 1981; 1984).

In particular, I observed what a dominant role formal models played on these units. It is on this topic that I shall focus, presenting some of my observations of the use and misuse of such models and trying to differentiate between the purposes for which they appear helpful and those for which they are inadequate.

| Formal Models

Formal models played a central role both practically and conceptually on these units. New nurses, of whom there were many, were provided checklists of the types of procedures, medications, and surgeries their patients would have. After two months, six months, and one year, these new nurses were painstakingly evaluated in peer review against the job descriptions that were organized around the nursing process model: assessment, planning, intervention, and evaluation. Nurses who had been there for a longer time were evaluated annually against the job description or whenever they sought promotion to a higher position.

Nursing care plans were a serious priority on these units. They consisted of printed "Standards of Care" for the major types of surgeries treated on the units. For example, there was a standard of care for "major abdominal surgery" in which the typical types of problems encountered by patients having these surgeries were listed with "expected outcomes" and "nursing orders." Progress notes of the nursing care plans were organized following Weed's (1970) Problem-Oriented Record System model under the acronym SOAP (Subjective, Objective, Assessment, and Plan). Finally, formal procedure manuals, which spell out how to do procedures such as hyperalimentation or dressing changes, or protocols, which spell out the rules to follow for particular situations, such as a code blue, were also in active use on these units.

Before exploring some of the uses and misuses of these models that I observed, let's first consider what I mean by formal models. Formal models are *explicit* statements composed of *elements* that have been selected *out of a larger context* and *reordered* to make a *new whole.* They are *representations,* and in this sense are abstract, appearing most often in written form. They put into fixed statements meanings that are often implicit, unstated, and loosely interpreted. Clifford Geertz discusses two senses in which cultural patterns are "models": models *of* reality and models *for* reality (1973:93). This distinction applies to the functions of formal models as well. Formal models provide a model *of* reality, an abstract representation like a map, at the same time as they provide a model *for* reality, a standard of how reality should be. They both reflect and direct.

227

Formal Models as Maps: A Way of Compensating for a Lack of Practical Mastery

Formal models can function much like a map for those who lack practical experience and mastery in a given area. Such persons, or groups of persons, need to be furnished with guides that outline a repertoire of rules that can be applied or a role that can be performed (Bourdieu, 1977:2). In this way, the formal model is a substitute for practical mastery, much as a map serves the outsider who lacks the first-hand knowledge of a native. This lack of practical mastery can apply, as I observed, both to a profession as a whole, such as in a situation of cultural change, or to individuals who lack personal experience and practical knowledge.

For the professional group lacking mastery, formal models can be a means of *institutionalizing new behaviors and attitudes*. They can provide a blueprint for change, specifying new behaviors and attitudes nurse leaders wish to be developed. Behaviors that were once hidden, unofficial, or rare can be made official, legitimate, and normative through formal models.

> *Example:* The job descriptions used on the units I studied were very carefully written by nurse leaders and representatives over a three-year period. The authors sought to make some nursing behaviors more visible, such as nursing assessments, so that nurses could receive more credit for them. They sought to legitimate some of nursing's unrecognized power and to make nurses formally accountable for their work. In addition, they sought to make some of nursing's occasional, haphazard behavior, such as attention or lack of attention to psychosocial issues, more consistent and normative. Finally, they sought to introduce new behaviors, such as research, more prominently. They used a formal model, consisting of very specifically writ-

ten job descriptions, to introduce these behaviors as new norms and general standards against which all nurses would be evaluated. This, in fact, took place while I was observing the units.

In spite of conspicuous results achieved from the use of such models, several danger signals cannot be overlooked. The formal model can easily come to be viewed as complete and an end in itself rather than a means to an end. The model, which is an abstraction, is sometimes approached as very real and concrete; it becomes reified. For example, nurses were sometimes told that they had realized "100 percent or 98 percent of the job description." There was a tendency to equate fulfilling of the job description with being a good and complete nurse, even though job descriptions cannot begin to capture the myriad of dimensions of good nursing.

Further, since job descriptions are written as statements of behavior that can be quantifiably evaluated, important aspects of nursing, such as caring and sensitivity, that cannot be easily measured are almost inherently eliminated. Additionally, one of the trademarks of expert practice is its contingent nature — i.e., action is taken depending on the *particular* rather than typical situation at hand. By its very nature this flexibility and situatedness cannot be predicted in a formal model.

Another danger is that, while formal models such as these job descriptions may pave the way for new behaviors that allow for more autonomy for nurses, once these behaviors are mastered, the spelling out of autonomy becomes a contradiction in terms.* Rather, much

---

*I am grateful to Dr. Elizabeth Colson for this idea.

autonomy derives from the unstated and unspecified, the freedom to realize goals through a variety of means.

For the individual lacking mastery, formal models can serve as *a substitute for personal knowledge and experience*. Much as these models can compensate for lack of mastery within a professional group, so they can also compensate for the inadequate knowledge and experience of individual nurses. They are essential teaching guides, as they spell out what to do in situations in which the performer has had no prior experience. By breaking down activities into elements and providing pertinent rules, they permit inexperienced nurses to undertake a new role and act with relative safety, or so it is hoped. Standards of Care, procedure manuals, and protocols fall into this category.

> *Example:* Some of the experienced nurses I observed had participated in writing up Standards of Care for the major surgeries treated on the units, such as mastectomies, major abdominal surgeries, or hernia repair. On the basis of their experience and relevant literature they wrote down, step by step, the typical problems and the activities to be taken in the care of patients who have undergone a particular type of surgery. The Standards point out what signs to look for, what typical problems to expect (such as infection or pain) as well as what steps to take in the face of a particular problem. A nurse who is new or who is a "float nurse" can read these standards and *generally* figure out what to do in a situation.

It is very important to note that these Standards of Care and similar models become the guides of behavior not only for the novice or "float nurse" but also for more experienced nurses. Such models, as well as personnel, become the carriers of culture and the standards of care (Gordon, 1981). In other words, the formal models are often teaching guides and play an essential role in the socialization and evaluation of nurses. To some extent, they replace the ongoing judgment of nursing personnel.

There are clearly some benefits to this externalization of knowledge. Putting nursing knowledge into a written form that a newcomer can read and act on allows the formal model to substitute for nursing personnel that may be absent. It extends nursing expertise when nurse experts are gone. It allows for interchangeability of nurses; a variety of nurses, for instance, can step into the same role and perform relatively safely rather than the knowledge residing with only a few nurses. In the face of nursing turnover, nursing shortages, and lack of recognition of what years of experience can teach, this interchangeability often has a very high value in the hospital setting.

This written documentation of nursing knowledge also provides a backup memory for more epxerienced nurses as well as newcomers. In fact, many expert nurses found the Standards of Care helpful as a safety net in case they forgot something – a distinct possibility as they typically had so many things on their mind simultaneously. With a backup list they did not have to keep everything in their heads.

One danger inherent in this use of formal models as compensation for lack of mastery, however, is that it does not differentiate between the beginner and the competent, proficient, or expert nurse. This lack of differentiation can be insulting and inappropriate.

Example: The nursing care plans consist both of Standards of Care for typical problems that are identified by individual nurses and of nursing orders based on these identified problems. For example, a patient who has been identified as depressed will have a nursing order requiring the nurse on duty to check on the patient every X number of hours and to provide that patient the opportunity to "ventilate" his/her feelings. This order does not take into account the patients who may not want to "ventilate" with a particular nurse. But that is not the only problem. To paraphrase one experienced nurse's reactions to these orders: "I resent being told to go in and visit a depressed patient. I would do that on my own, out of my own concern. I don't need to be legislated to do so."

Nursing orders, geared toward the typical situation, are not directed to the particular needs and desires of the individual patient nor to the particularities of the nurse. They work better for stable patient care situations and are less suited for the majority of acute and rapidly changing patient care situations. Further, nursing orders generally assume very little knowledge on the part of the performer. For those who already know what to do and who can distinguish fine nuances in patient situations not accounted for in the Standards of Care, the nursing orders can be insulting.

Similarly, formal models, usually organized on the basis of the lowest common denominator, can be alienating and unchallenging to those with the greatest expertise. In fact, formal models are impersonal, taking a "nurse is a nurse" approach. Nursing, in trying to differentiate nursing expertise, to move beyond obedience to medical orders, and to become more autonomous and accountable can ill afford to reinforce impersonality and mere obedience by adding more rules that tend to restrict judgment.

There is a further danger of spelling out nursing behavior in an explicit, elemental fashion. Much as formal models can break down a complex situation into manageable bits, they can break it down into so many bits it can become unmanageable. While trying to be absolutely thorough, to take nothing for granted, formal models can become exhaustive lists that prove overwhelming for nurses who encounter them.

Example: Nursing orders for some procedures on patient care run several pages. Teaching plans for wound care, written out in a step by step form, often left even competent nurses feeling overwhelmed and insecure. When several nurses repeatedly complained of difficulty following the care plan for changing the dressing of a patient the head nurse went to check the care plan and dressing herself. She found that she too was intimidated and bewildered by the pages of notes. It took her several readings to recognize familiar procedures and to figure out what to do, which in the end was not that difficult. She was not surprised that both newer and more veteran nurses were overwhelmed by the stream of proscribed behaviors.

In other words, spelling out activities in too much detail can lead to a sense of more rather than less complexity. In philosophy, this is called the problem of infinite regress (Dreyfus, 1979): the fact that each time one spells out clearly what is taken for granted, one faces still another set of assumptions that need to be spelled out.

Guide Through Difficult Terrain In their reduction and explicitness, formal models can provide a guide through difficult and overwhelming emotional terrain, a compass for direction. In this way they offer a means for coping with difficult emotional situations.

Example: A new nurse had her first encounter with a dying patient and was somewhat overwhelmed by the experience. In a patient conference held on her behalf, she and others were presented Kübler-Ross's model of the stages of grief. Both the patient's and the nurse's respective stages were identified by the group. The new nurse clearly gained better understanding of the situation as a result.

The danger here, however, is in providing explanations and means for handling complex situations that verge on oversimplification and closing off.

> *Example:* In the same example as above, the nurse was identified as being in one of Kübler-Ross's stages of grief called "bargaining." She was identified as actively negotiating for more hope for the patient. Having spoken to her and watched her involvement I felt there was a great deal more to her feelings than this and that it was a gross simplification, a packaging and a dismissal of much of her experience, to so quickly pigeonhole her into this "stage."

Thus, one sees the other side of the coin. By reducing a vast kaleidoscope of dimensions into a selected number of variables in a model, formal models can squelch and tame the complexity of actual situations. Sometimes this simplification is desired, but sometimes complexity is essential. Particularly in sensitive situations like caring for dying patients, formal models can close off deep understanding rather than open it, thus providing a false sense of certainty and control rather than ambiguity and vulnerable involvement. When helping patients, involvement and openness to complexity are sometimes critical. The reductionism of formal models can then go both ways: it simplifies and orders, but when taken too far or used in the wrong situations, it can obscure and exclude important dimensions of the situation.

Formal Models as a Basis for Consensus and Standardization

We've seen how formal models can function as maps or substitutes for knowledge. A second major use is for them to serve as a basis for conformity and a statement of the ideal. These models can be a guide for normative behavior and can help standardize behavior in the face of diversity or lack of shared understandings.

Social groups require some consensus on how to behave and what is important to meet their needs both as individuals and as a group. The most common source of this consensus is through shared life experiences — time spent together. Typically, social groups that share life experiences also share a large stock of intersubjective meanings (Taylor, 1971) that all participants understand on an implicit level. The likelihood for consensus and understanding among the members about practices, interpretations, and values is great, the result of repeated social interaction.

But what of groups that do not share a history, groups that not only come from diverse backgrounds but have and expect to work together only briefly? Or what of groups who face cultural change, such that the background they shared is no longer relevant? In situations like these, formal models can provide the basis for consensus, a blueprint or standard for behavior that all can follow. Thus, where one cannot rely on an *implicit* basis of understanding that comes from shared experience and knowledge, one can turn to *explicit* understanding, provided by formal models that describe behaviors that all are expected to see and follow. In this important way, formal models substitute for a background of shared practices and meanings.

> *Example:* The job descriptions on the units were carefully written so that they could serve as a model for new behaviors. But they were clearly more than a model or a map. They were a new standard, a universal standard against which all nurses were measured. To make this possible, the job descriptions were formally written as behavioral statements that could be quantitatively evaluated, such as "communicates a rationale to the patient."

The novelty of many solicited behaviors indicated the lack of a background of shared understanding. Nurses, in many cases, simply did not have a history of carrying out these behaviors. Lacking a common and experiential background that could serve as group ideals or norms, the job descriptions furnished a standard to which people from a variety of backgrounds were expected to conform. Nursing as a profession characterized by scientific, autonomous, accountable, rational practice was the ideal implied in the statements, and the behavioral statements — the model — were meant to solicit this ideal in behavior.

It could be argued that greater understanding is made possible by making meanings, expectations, and values explicit, that doing so allows for greater clarity, that even in the presence of shared understandings it is still preferable to spell things out explicitly. But, while explicit statements are important substitutes for tacit understanding, they are not the same thing. Formal explicit statements fix meaning and do not allow for nuances of interpretation the way tacit understanding does. Stating meanings explicitly also takes time. The kind of communication that can take place among familiars, the one look or the one word that "speak a thousand words," is far from possible when one lacks a background of familiarity. Even if one has it and one tries to spell out those "thousand words," one runs into problems; only certain things can be put into words. It is worth nothing that it took a good part of three years to write the job descriptions (and design a new clinical ladder); it also took a few years to write the Standards of Care.

Another concern about relying on formal models as standards and the basis of consensus and evaluation is the danger of demanding excessive conformity. It is very easy to pursue only the narrow options for behavior specified in the model and to expect constricting conformity from the actors.

Misuses of Models

As outlined earlier, formal models can be very powerful and even essential in some situations. But because of what may verge on an excessive and unquestioning reliance on formal models in nursing communities and in American society in general, it is important to consider more fully some of the ways in which formal models are misused. Here, too, I draw on a few observed examples.

Standardizing the Contingent and Substituting Rules for Judgment

Nurses are faced with many complex and multiple decisions as they provide care. Writing out protocols could circumvent some judgment by standardizing activities in a safe, albeit perhaps inefficient, way, but protocols and formulas cannot substitute for judgment in some situations and the understanding of the situation that is necessary for that judgment.

> *Example:* On the units I observed, new nurses learned the role of charge nurse after seven and eight weeks on the unit, first with supervision, later without. Several nurses had initial and continual difficulties handling the multiple demands of the role. In an effort to alleviate these difficulties, one nurse worked on a protocol for the charge role, writing out what a charge nurse is supposed to do. While this master list was a comprehensive reminder of things to remember, it could not prioritize situation by situation, demand by demand; it could not assess relevance or antici-

pate the problems before they came; it could not prescribe interpretations for the new nurse, such as tell her which nurses at a particular time needed help. It could not make the nurse "see the unit as a whole," a perception so necessary for effective charge duties.

Similarly, nursing report proved to be a difficult activity for the new nurse to learn. Efforts to standardize what was presented in report were occasionally pursued. But a good report can never be standardized because the essence of a good report is passing on only the essential information as well as anticipating problems for the new shift. For this reason, vital signs, for example, have no fixed importance from case to case; in some cases they are crucial information, in others of little importance. The same is true of diet, intravenous solution, "intakes and outputs," and other information in the report. A good report selects what is most important to know for the care of a patient, a *selection*, not a *predetermined* set of information. And in order to select, the nurse must understand the patient's general situation.

In both of these examples, the nurses involved knew well the difference between a good report and a bad one, a good charge role performance and a bad one. But I think in the face of pressure to speed up the grasp of the new nurses, a turn was made to formal models that, while helping, could never be the answer. Perhaps the answer would come in knowing that a good grasp of the situation was necessary to give a good report or to be in charge, and that maybe more time should be given before new nurses are asked to perform such duties alone.

Formal models cannot circumvent judgment. Although standards of care have garnered nursing knowledge and formulated procedural steps, they are geared to the typical situation — the average patient, not a particular patient. It is still up to the individual nurse to recognize and interpret a situation as relevant.

Example: A standard care plan designates "pain" as a typical problem of postsurgical general abdominal surgical patients. It does not and cannot, however, specify what constitutes a problem level of pain, particularly given the range of patient responses. Obviously some pain is experienced by all patients. But at what point does it constitute a problem? One must make an interpretation. Postoperative pain management requires astute judgment so that the patient is neither undermedicated nor overmedicated. The result I observed is that newcomers who as yet had little sense of the range of tolerable levels of discomfort and pain sometimes misjudged the need for pain medication. Here one sees that formal models are only as good as their users.

Relying Excessively on Formal Models and Rules to Achieve Order and Control

Procedures, standards, and rules provide order and guides to situations and a general assurance of safe activity. They are, however, no guarantee of "quality care," as it is often alluded to.

Example I: The units often experienced great stress trying to absorb and teach large numbers of new nurses how to provide good, safe care. The nurse leaders desperately wanted to provide "quality nursing care" and stressed repeatedly the need to write out care plans and histories, to document correctly, and to meet other standards. I think that the quality of care given on the unit sometimes became equated with meeting these formal standards. Yet these external standards, while intended to guarantee safe care, could in no way capture the quality of patient care actually given by individual nurses. In fact, many nurses, when pinched for time, pushed care plans into the back seat. Some complained of not being recognized for managing the unit during stressed times or for giving good care to patients while short-staffed, that the circumstances around their care were not attended to in the formal care plans. It sometimes appeared to some that what mattered most was the documentation and meeting of formal rules.

Example II: If one studies the job descriptions and the actual content of peer review evaluations in this setting, one finds much emphasis placed on writing skills of the nurse, e.g., taking and writing a good nursing history, care plan, and SOAP charting. These more formalizable traits become associated with being a good nurse whereas traits and activities such as caring, timing, and early recognition of patient changes get overlooked.

Following rules, while essential for the novice and inexperienced, provides only one type of order and by no means the best. One can also have order without recourse to rules (Dreyfus, 1979), order based on an assessment of the particular situation in terms of the particular intents and concerns and skills of the performer. This order derives from the matching of concerns, interpretation of a situation, and action that is appropriate to the performers and situations and is grasped in a holistic way. Behavior may be streamlined, since what is unnecessary can be deleted; this is not the case in formal models.

When order and "quality care" become equated with following the rules, as I think has sometimes occurred in the settings I observed, one can even say that the competent level of skill, as described in the Dreyfus model of skill acquisition, has become defined as the ideal (Gordon, 1982). Standards geared to experts would look very different than formal, explicit rules. Further, formal models can provide a false sense of control and certainty; they may provide the *basis* for safe care but not necessarily the best care. This difference must not be forgotten.

Mystification

A further danger of excessive reliance on formal models and formal language is mystification. Speech and thought become sloganized and formalized to such an extent that very narrow and unquestioned discourse takes place, obscuring the complexity of the actual situation for the actors. This often serves a necessary function for nurses in complex, high-demand situations, but the dangers must be foreseen and the limits understood. There is also a danger that people *think* they know what they mean when in fact they don't, or that the meanings become so general as to be meaningless.

> *Example:* Having followed two expert nurses for over two months each, I wrote up my observations noting, in particular, how the two excellent nurses practiced nursing so differently. One was a very active presence, a force to be dealt with; the other worked rather like an invisible helpful force who understated her presence rather than emphasized it. In discussing with me what was special about these nurses, a nurse leader who knew them both well noted that they were both excellent at "psycho-social skills." Nevertheless, lumping both of these nurses into a general characterization of good psycho-social skills seemed to mark and obscure the subtle skills of these nurses and to perform a disservice to the appreciation of excellent nursing. The term "psycho-social" has come to take on so much meaning it can become almost meaningless, a term used to describe either how nurses interact with patients or patient concerns that are clearly not biological. Such frequent and general use of this important concept leaves it almost bereft of meaning and subtlety.

| Summary

Since the uses of formal models in nursing appear to be well appreciated, let me summarize some of the *dangers* of excessive reliance on formal models: (1) reification: equating the model with reality; (2) an eclipse or a devaluing of traits that cannot be formalized; (3) legislation of behavior that contradicts the goal of nursing autonomy; (4) alienation and lack of challenge to more experienced nurses in favor of inexperienced; (5) spelling out so much it overwhelms rather than helps; (6) oversimplification of complex situations; (7) demand for excessive conformity: using the same standard for all people may demand excessive conformity to a particular set of standards; (8) insensitivity to nuances in patient situations and, in particular, nurses: formal statements are geared towards the typical rather than the particular; (9) confusion between following rules and the need for judgment; and (10) mystification: speech becomes so sloganized it becomes trivial and narrow in meaning.

What can we learn from this research? First, that the functions of formal models depend on the situation and the intents of the users. Some of the characteristics of formal models — their reductionism, their elemental approach, their explicitness, their objectivity — are exactly what is desired in some situations. In others, however, they work against the goals and intents of the users, such as indirectly restricting autonomy among nurses by legislating nursing action through "nursing orders" or elaborate job descriptions.

It is not only important that formal models be used with discretion, but that they and their features not be overvalued in favor or in eclipse of traits that are not formalizable, such as the relational, the contingent, the nonverbal, the holistic, or the intuitive. This danger is well fueled by the dominant epistemological tradition in our society and a model of science that thrives on formalization and formal models.

Nursing, in its bid for professional status, autonomy, greater effectiveness in patient care, and greater legitimacy must be wary of overreliance and idealization of traits that nursing has formerly lacked, excessively relying on formal models as the way to nursing's goals. While nursing must cope with the constraints presented by medicine and bureaucracy, nurses can ill afford to create new chains themselves, particularly in the name of freedom and growth. Let formal models in many cases be regarded as training wheels, essential for the first safe rides, unnecessary and limiting once replaced by greater skill. Let not reality be confused with the model. And let us not forget that the model is a tool, not a mirror.*

*The author wishes to thank the many nurses who generously participated in this study and Dr. Esther Lucile Brown and Dr. Patricia Benner for their intellectual and editorial contributions.

243

Implementation of Staff Nurse III at El Camino Hospital

by Ann Huntsman, R.N., M.S.; Janet Reiss Lederer, R.N., M.S.; and Elaine M. Peterman, R.N., B.S.

As Benner has said, "Recognition, reward and retention of the experienced nurse in positions of direct clinical practice — along with the documentation and adequate description of their practice — are the first steps in improving the quality of patient care."[1] At El Camino Hospital in Mountain View, California, we wanted to establish a clinical ladder that would acknowledge advanced clinical nursing practice. We describe here how such a program was developed and implemented.

A task force was formed that represented a cross-section of professional nurses: staff nurses, nursing instructor, nursing coordinator, head nurse, and the director of education and training. The co-director of the AMICAE* Project was retained as consultant. Two task

[1]Benner, Patricia, "From Novice to Expert," *Am. J. Nursing* 82:402–407. March 1982.

*AMICAE, Achieving Methods of Intra-professional Consensus, Assessment, and Evaluation, was a federally funded evaluation study of new graduate nurses from seven schools of nursing in the San Francisco Bay Area. In this study, researchers also observed and described the practice of expert nurse clinicians.

force members had participated in AMICAE project interviews; they had described experiences in which their nursing interventions had made a difference.

We were enthusiastic about an approach that involved experienced nurses' descriptions of clinical situations in which they made a difference. After a review of the exemplars of skilled nursing performance identified in the AMICAE project, the task force built the Staff Nurse III (SN III) description on that framework, and part of the SN III's documentation for peer review was to include written exemplars representing his or her best work. (Staff Nurse I is the entry level position, and the nurse advances to Staff Nurse II after one year (6 months for the baccalaureate nurse) of employment. Nursing process is the basis for the R.N. job description at El Camino Hospital.

Over a four-month period, the task force came together in one-day workshops facilitated by the consultant. We brainstormed ideas and engaged in much discussion around issues of developing a credible process for recognition of excellent nursing practice. One issue was how to build a process that would ensure sustained practice once this had been recognized. Another issue was the probability that many nurses would not qualify for promotion to SN III. This was resolved after lengthy discussion of the need to reward those nurses whose practice was more advanced than that of their colleagues.

The major components of the SN III description included general requirements and four areas of responsibility: to client, for advancement of nursing knowledge, for development of self and others, and to clinical unit and organization.

At two different intervals a draft of the SN III description was sent to all head nurses, nursing coordinators,

245

and staff development instructors for review and comment, and their recommendations were incorporated into the final SN III description. In a one-day workshop, those nurses selected to be on the two peer review committees were oriented to the Staff Nurse III application process and their responsibilities in that process.

Peer Review Process

Peer review, the method used to evaluate and promote candidates to the SN III classification, provides an objective means for (1) providing evaluation feedback about clinical practice to staff nurse III candidates; (2) recognizing the clinician who has advanced skills and knowledge; and (3) promoting a system that encourages professional assessment and accountability.

Members of the peer review committee(s) are appointed by the assistant administrator, nursing, for a minimum of one year. Appointments allow for both continuity and change in committee members. Each committee is composed of a nursing coordinator, one head nurse, a staff development instructor who acts as a facilitator, and three staff nurse IIIs from differing clinical areas. This committee composition provides for a diverse, well-rounded approach to the appraisal of the candidate's nursing practice.

The committee(s) meet quarterly to review SN III candidates. The only data used in making recommendations regarding promotion are the candidate's profile folder and the interview. Thus, the more clearly a profile folder reflects the quality of the candidate's nursing practice, the more effective the committee can be in making its recommendation. Contents of the folder include:

Application form indicating candidate's compliance with general requirements and documentation of educational experience.

Copy of last performance appraisal.

Self-evaluation of performance in each area of responsibility identified in the job description and a description of professional goals, short- and long-term.

Evaluation by two sponsors, head nurse or assistant head nurse and a peer, of the candidate's choice in the areas of responsibility identified in the job description.

Narrative description of a clinical situation that reflects the candidate's best work (a narratively written exemplar).

Written evidence of involvement in committee work or special projects.

Items that reflect the quality of the candidate's work such as nursing care plans, nurse's notes, project work.

Letter of reference from colleague of candidate's choice (optional).

Preceding the interview, each committee member independently reviews the candidate's folder in the interests of objectivity and reduction of bias. Contents of the folder and review impressions remain confidential.

During the folder review, committee members begin to formulate and note questions they wish to ask the candidate in the interview. To promote an organized and consistent approach to folder review, a form was developed for use as a worksheet for recording comments and questions, noting impressions, and the like. This worksheet is used by the individual reviewer as a reference before and during the interview process.

The candidate is asked to participate in a 45-minute interview as a part of the application for promotion. A staff development instructor facilitates the group process prior to and during the interview and also during the discussion phase after the interview has been completed. We have found it important that each member of the interviewing team ask the candidate at least one question during the interview, since candidates have been known to interpret silence on the part of any one member as being a negative judgment.

We have attempted to create an ambience of comfort by choosing an informal interview site with comfortable chairs, couch, and small table. Coffee is offered. The interview is started on time. A chair is provided outside the interviewing room in case the candidate arrives earlier than the specified time.

Once the candidate has been seated for the interview, introductions are made. Each interviewer gives her or his name, title, and specialty area. The staff development instructor then explains the interview process to the candidate in a warm, friendly manner. Since candidates are often nervous during the interview, we try to provide a supportive environment through our conversational and nonverbal interactions with the candidate. A reference to the positive aspects of the profile folder is always stressed during the explanation of the interview process. The candidate is given ample time to respond to questions and comments and is encouraged to seek clarification of the questions and reactions to responses. The applicant is also asked to relate a clinical narrative that further exemplifies ability to perform at an SN III level. The story should demonstrate both the quality of nursing practice and involvement with clients. The interviewers may request clarification of aspects of the clinical narrative or ask probing questions to further determine the candidate's level of practice.

Here are three examples of such narratives:

| Clinical Situation Narrative

Kathy Brown, R.N.

I was assigned 3 uncomplicated patients on pms in CCU and was asked to transfer another patient to 4W at 4 pm. Days had been too busy. I planned to assess my 3 patients after a quick check of my transfer. I had cared for Mr. M. over the weekend and felt I knew him well enough to just stick my head in to say, "Hi, I'll be back later," but something was not right. He was slumped to the side and was breathing hard. His color was OK, though. I lingered and confirmed that he was anticipating transfer at 4 pm. The transfer summary was written, papers ready, bags packed — "just wheel him down the hall." I shifted my plan to quick check the other three (BP and rhythm stable, no pain) and settled in to read the progress notes to learn what had transpired since yesterday. Besides a turnover of physicians from the weekend, there was not much new. Pulmonary edema had pretty well resolved and an MI had been ruled out. I decided to assess Mr. M. more carefully and wished I didn't have three other "real patients." I mentioned to my AHN that I was concerned about Mr. M. and asked her to look in on others and to arrange to delay the transfer. I found vital signs unchanged, except for respirations up to 30. Lungs had minimal rales, face waxen, trunk cyanotic, urinary output poor and a feeling of weakness. No specific pain.

With little clinical evidence and more of a "gut feeling," I telephoned the primary physician to report my observation and the subtle changes. She was unavailable, but I reached the cardiologist who agreed ABGs were in order, and additional lab work was drawn, though today's chest X-ray showed an improvement. He agreed to temporarily hold up transfer. I conferred with the AHN and asked to be relieved of one patient. This patient was exhibiting more than the usual signs of transfer anxiety, but I had trouble putting my finger on it.

I called the primary physician again, with the abnormal lab results to support my "gut feeling." The physician arrived shortly to assess the patient, and the possibilities of pulmonary embolism, pleural effusion with renal failure were studied as I prepared Mr. M. for thoracentesis and pulmonary angiograms before I left at 1 AM.

Mr. M. followed a rocky course with several uncertain diagnoses which have not been easily treated. These are the difficulties one learns to live with in critical care. The rewards come when a particularly difficult physician thanks you for your acuity in assessing the patient and acting appropriately.

Clinical Situation Narrative

Lucy Ann Nomura, R.N.

Mr. Smith was a 70-year-old man who had a bowel resection for cancer. He was transferred to the surgical unit from the intensive care unit on his third postoperative day. On his first day on our unit, I helped care for him and found him to be pleasant and cooperative. On this particular day, I was his primary nurse. During the night he had projectile vomiting. After the morning abdominal X-ray showed fluid in the bowel, a naso-gastric tube was inserted. My initial assessment that morning showed the vital signs to be unremarkable (BP 110/70; T. 100; AP 100 and slightly irregular; R. 20). His abdomen was softly distended and somewhat tender to touch. Also, I noted his slow affect which I thought was *not* due to lack of sleep.

When his wife came to visit, she confirmed my suspicions by asking if I had given Mr. Smith some medication to make him drowsy. Since I believe in the importance of keeping family members informed, I re-assured Mrs. Smith that the doctor and I were aware of the change in her husband's mental state and told her about the planned course of treatment.

I had already expressed my concern to Mr. Smith's doctor earlier that morning. The doctor thought that Mr. Smith was just dehydrated and that an increase in I.V. fluids would improve his condition clinically.

In the early afternoon, there was a slight change in vital signs (BP 100/60; T. 100; AP 102; R. 20) and he was more difficult to arouse. Along with an intuitive feeling of something seriously wrong with Mr. Smith, I remembered an article about the insidious onset of septicemia in older people—there may or may not be a slightly lowered BP, low-grade fever, and sometimes the most noticeable sign of trouble might be a change in the mental state. I again called the doctor to update him on the latest vital signs, and tell him about the low urine output despite increased I.V. fluids. Although I could not point to any overt sign, my persistence and obvious concern for Mr. Smith brought the doctor back to the hospital. Upon my suggestion, he inserted a CVP line and ordered a stat CBC. Later that day, Mr. Smith was taken back to the operating room for emergency surgery, based on an elevated white blood count and an increasing lack of response.

The following day, his doctor told me that he found a leakage of the anastamosis site with resultant peritonitis. Then the doctor thanked me for my perceptive nursing care and thoughtful concern on the previous day.

Clinical Situation Narrative

Janet Crowley, R.N.

My patient was a six-week-old, rather hefty boy, who had been operated on the evening before for pyloric stenosis. The postoperative orders from the physician stated: "Wait two hours, then offer 2 ounces of karo water, followed by 2 ounces ½-strength breast milk, then 2 ounces full strength breast milk, then increase to breast feeding ad lib." The child tolerated his feedings well the evening after surgery and by 11 PM had taken 7–8 ounces of fluid. At 12 AM the child voided for the first time since admission, took 2 ounces of breast milk, and vomited the entire feeding, plus. Throughout the night the child continued to vomit all feedings taken. At 6 AM the child had vomited slightly more than he had taken in on the night shift. The child's surgeon was notified and instructions were given to keep trying oral feedings and notify the child's pediatrician if the child were unable to retain fluids.

My assessment of the child was that he was alert, skin turgor good, and mucous membranes slightly moist. The child voided as I was taking his temperature. I assessed that the child was not currently dehydrated; however, with frequent vomiting and poor intake, the child could quickly become so.

In my experience with children with pyloric stenosis, I have found that most children have difficulty tolerating 2 ounces at one feeding. I have found that patients much better tolerated frequent very small feedings. My nursing care plan was to start with ½ ounce karo water every 30 minutes. When the child tolerated three feedings at each step, I slowly advanced his diet. After each feeding I placed the child in an infant seat on his right side. At the end of my shift the child was tolerating 1 ounce full-strength breast milk every hour. He had taken and retained 150 cc. and had vomited only about 20 cc. The child did well on the evening shift and was discharged the next day.

I choose this example because I feel it best shows the nursing process. The child was quickly restored to health without any unnecessary procedures and cost. The child did not get dehydrated and did not require any intravenous fluids.

Once the interviewers have explored all aspects necessary to reach a decision, the interview is ended. The committee members then reflect on the interview and, through consensus, submit a written recommendation for classification to the assistant administrator for nursing who makes the final decision and notifies the candidate in writing within 10 working days following the interview. If the assistant administrator has any questions or concerns about the decisions after she has reviewed the folder and the written comments from the interviewing group, she meets with members of the committee for more input.

As might have been expected, some "chinks" have surfaced in the interviewing system. One is bias, and the other is the problem of reaching consensus.

It is impossible to select only those interviewing team members who have no personal knowledge of the candidate, since candidates seeking the SN III position have usually interfaced with some of the interviewers either on hospital committees or as peers on the clinical unit. Because of this, an element of bias (either positive or negative) may enter into the decision. During the discussion following the interview, these biases are addressed so that the interviewers are aware of the variables that enter the decision. Since six nurses are interviewing the candidate, we have found that bias is reduced by the ability of the group to consider opinions of those members who don't know the candidate personally. Whenever the committee has identified bias as a barrier in decision-making, another group is asked to review the candidate's folder and to conduct an interview. Decision is by consensus; all members must agree with the recommendation.

The peer review interview is conducted for the new applicant to SN III and every other year for renewal of that status. On the alternate years, a profile folder is the only necessary item in the peer review process.

Impact on the Organization

The reason for asking the nurse to present her or his case for promotion both orally and in writing was because it was anticipated that some clinicians might present a better case one way or the other. Occasionally, this has turned out to be the case; a nurse might present an outstanding written case but because of anxiety would not perform well in the interview, or vice versa. But usually the written profile has been predictive of the oral presentation.

The problems in the written profile related to the candidate's written presentation of her or his practice, the manager's performance appraisal, and, to a lesser degree, the peer sponsor's presentation of the candidate's work. In general, nurses proved reluctant to, as they put it, "blow their own horn" or "sell" themselves, both verbally and in writing. They frequently wrote about their practice in global terms or parroted the job description without giving specific examples of behaviors that substantiated the described level of performance. When addressing the matter of responsibility to clients, a surprising number of candidates wrote in the third person. Peer sponsors, too, were often not specific in describing the nursing practice of the candidate.

However, this has improved markedly as the number of SN IIIs has increased. Nurses who have been promoted now coach nurses who are preparing their cases. One organized group of professional nurses in the hospital has established a formal class to help nurses prepare for clinical promotion. At first there was suspicion that the number of SN IIIs would be limited and that managerial agendas would outweigh the professional merits of the nurse's case but now, with a two-year history, the nurses are confident that if they meet the requirements they will be promoted. They speak today in the first person and carefully select actual episodes from their own practice. A side benefit is that nurses are talking about their own practice and are receiving acknowledgement for advanced clinical judgment.

The strongest resource for the SN III applicant in profile folder preparation and the interview process are the SN IIIs who are members of the peer review committee(s). Other resources are their head nurse, assistant head nurse, and/or staff development instructor.

Performance appraisal issues, again, were largely that of the manager's failure to document comprehensive and specific descriptions of the candidate's level of practice. The format of the appraisal did not follow that of the SN III job description. Often, the performance appraisal offered the committee no supportive resource upon which to base its recommendation.

The peer review process has heightened awareness of the need for specific descriptions of nursing practice in the performance appraisal. Head nurses on the peer review committee have provided direction to their peers. In addition, the assistant administrator for nursing has conducted small group workshops to refine performance appraisal skills.

Summary

It has been a very rewarding experience to see excellent nurses finally being recognized and rewarded for their level of practice. For the individual promoted to SN III, it has been professionally enriching and validating to be so honored and to explain to inquiring patients what SN III means on the name pin. Financially, the promotion means a 5 percent increase in salary.

Interestingly, SN IIIs who have been appointed to the peer review committee are adamant about upholding the criteria and standards of the SN III program. Maintaining the quality of the process is very important to them.

Several instances have occurred in which SN IIIs have demonstrated increased awareness of their influence and impact on nursing practice in their work area. This includes the informal communication among staff nurses as well as the formal occurrences when an SN III is acting as a preceptor, resource nurse, or unit representative on a nursing committee. Frequently an SN III will coach one of her colleagues in preparing an application for promotion.

We believe our experience with describing and formalizing the promotion to SN III* has acknowledged the proficient nurse and has laid the foundation for the exciting challenge of the next phase: describing the *expert* nurse clinician.†

*The Staff Nurse III description, application, and peer review process are available through the Nursing Department at El Camino Hospital.

†The authors wish to thank Ruth Colavecchio, co-director of the AMICAE Project and consultant in the early development of this program.

Focus on Excellence

by Jeanette Ullery, R.N., M.S.N., Director of Staff Development, St. Luke's Regional Medical Center, Mountain States Tumor Institute, Boise, Idaho

There is much in the literature about the need to recognize and reward the staff nurse, yet so few examples of how recognition has been accomplished. At St. Luke's Regional Medical Center we believe we have developed a highly unusual and stimulating program that provides recognition as well as assists in the development of staff's clinical knowledge and in the continued striving for excellence in nursing practice.

In March 1982, a symposium entitled "Focus on Excellence" was arranged for our registered and licensed practical nurse staff; the sponsor — an appreciative patient and family — stipulated that we were to arrange a special nursing symposium that would contribute to the knowledge and skills of the majority of St. Luke's nursing staff. They contributed funds to reserve symposium space in a local convention center, lunch for all attendees, as well as an honorarium and expenses for the consultant. The same symposium was repeated on two consecutive days and was attended by 95 percent (232) of St. Luke's nursing staff and 13 Boise State University nursing faculty.

Planning began well in advance. The associate administrator for nursing appointed a program committee composed of staff nurses, head nurses, nursing administrators, staff development personnel, and the associate dean of the school of health sciences at Boise State University. The committee's task was to assist in the selection of the workshop topic, faculty, and a format that would provide both significant recognition of staff and a significant educational opportunity.

The theme was to recognize and reward excellence in nursing practice. The symposium faculty member was Patricia Benner, who had been involved in studies to identify the competencies of new graduates for over ten years. She applied the Dreyfus model of skill acquisition to nursing and, in so doing, offered guidelines for career and knowledge development in clinical nursing practice. The symposium offered opportunity for theory building and for individual exchange of practical knowledge. The result was an open recognition that the nurse was making important contributions in the daily world of work and in her profession.

Small group sessions of 10 to 15 staff nurses from different units met together with staff nurse facilitators to describe actual clinical situations where they learned something new or made a difference in the patient's care. The main function of the facilitators, who had eight hours of training prior to the program, was to start the nurses talking about their actual clinical practice in a narrative way that would include what they were thinking and expecting as well as what actually occurred. The facilitators encouraged the nurses to include in their description the "context" of the situation — i.e., what else was going on that had an impact on the situation.

259

Staff welcomed the opportunity to reflect on their excellence in nursing practice. They particularly valued the exchange of rich clinical experiences where nurses *had* made a difference in the patient's outcome; it seemed to provide them with the proverbial "shot in the arm." Some of the comments taken from the evaluations included: "provided unique opportunity for nurses at St. Luke's to be together"; "could relate with other colleagues that we never would get to know at work"; "made me feel proud to be a nurse"; "felt new surge of dedication to nursing"; and "liked supportive feeling among nurses." Instead of talking about problems to be solved or system deficits, they were actually taking time to review what they were doing well. When one nurse would give a story from her practice, other nurses would be stimulated to recall similar situations. In providing this unique opportunity for nurses to reflect on what they did well, the symposium opened up new areas of clinical learning. Growth in clinical judgment and skill can occur gradually over time and go unrecognized by the practitioner and his or her colleagues. The clinical knowledge development seminars allowed the nurses to notice and take credit for their accomplishments.

Since this symposium, we have continued to focus on excellence by encouraging staff to share paradigm cases. The same nurses who facilitated the small group sessions at the symposium now assist staff on the unit level to present outstanding clinical cases where they thought they made a difference.

These clinical episodes are more likely to deal with specific aspects of a patient situation rather than the entire length of stay. As a result, our nurses are beginning to have a shared background of patient care situations that they can discuss and compare when new cases are presented. This has proven to be an excellent way for staff to express feelings about patient care situations, to describe complicated patient care, and to enrich clinical knowledge of other staff by passing along hard-earned knowledge gained through experience.

We have had to increase the number of prepared facilitators in order to have one facilitator on each unit. Our criteria for selection of facilitators were that: (1) they had attended the Focus on Excellence symposium; (2) they were open, nonjudgmental persons respected by their peers; and (3) they were selected by the head nurse in conjunction with input from the already existing facilitator group.

It has been over a year since the symposium. We are still continuing the concept of crediting clinical knowledge and acknowledging situations in which the nurse made a difference or a special contribution to the patient's care. Not all staff are equally enthusiastic, but the majority find that their own practice is enhanced and that they find support for the difficult, risky decision making they do daily. We are continuing our individual unit clinical knowledge development seminars and are planning another symposium to provide opportunity for staff again to "focus on excellence."

Identification of the Skilled Performance of Master's Prepared Nurses as a Method of Curriculum Planning and Evaluation

by Mary V. Fenton, R.N., Dr. P.H.
  Associate Professor, University of Texas
  Medical Branch School of Nursing at Galveston

Two years ago the faculty of the graduate nursing program at the University of Texas Medical Branch in Galveston wanted to improve the evaluation of the clinical component of the graduate nursing program. We surveyed the clinical evaluation methods of 12 similar programs and found that they were experiencing some of the same kinds of general dissatisfaction with their current clinical evaluation methods. The program representatives shared their clinical evaluation instruments with us — instruments that had many of the same weaknesses that we identified in our own methods. After study and discussion, we concluded that our dissatisfaction with the evaluation tools stemmed from a lack of data and of agreement about the acceptable levels of skilled performance of master's prepared nurses in clinical settings.

This conclusion led to a redefinition of our original goal: we decided that we needed to identify the role, resources, demands, and constraints of individuals in actual practice settings before we could design instruments to evaluate the curriculum. The data on actual

role performance had not been systematically identified, compiled, and used as a basis for curriculum planning and evaluation. We concluded that knowledge of
the workaday world of the master's prepared nurse
would clarify those curriculum components that contribute to success in the master's role and would identify those areas where gaps exist and new knowledge is
needed.

The faculty wanted to know empirically what areas
of skilled performance were exhibited by master's prepared nurses in clinical settings. It was at this point
that, guided by the report of the AMICAE project (Benner et al., 1981), we determined that the domains of
expert practice as identified in that project could be
used as the basis for studying the practice of master's
prepared nurses. We felt that if these domains were
examples of expert practice, they, as well as additional
domains and competencies observed by faculty, could
be the basis for curriculum planning and evaluation.

A study was designed to identify the skilled performance of master's prepared nurses in a large state-refer-
ral, acute care health science center. The methodology
used in the AMICAE project was the model for this
study, and Dr. Benner served as a consultant. All faculty who teach in the graduate program served as interviewers and observers. Data collection methods
consisted of taped interviews of critical incidents and
participant observations of 34 master's prepared nurses
in the functional role categories of clinical specialist,
administrator, and educator. All three areas were
chosen because our program includes functional role
preparation in clinical practice (both clinical specialist
and practitioner), teaching, and management. All master's prepared nurses employed in the setting agreed to
participate in the study. They reflected a wide range of

experience and background. Seven were graduates of our own master's program; 17 were clinical specialists, 3 were in staff development and training roles, 9 were in administrative roles, 2 were head nurses, and 3 were staff nurses.

The analysis was divided into three parts: verification of the performance skills of expert nurses as reported in the AMICAE project; identification of new areas of skilled performance; and the emergence of five preliminary categories that have relevance for curriculum evaluation in the graduate nursing program. The critical incidents and participant observation data reflected all the domains identified by Benner as characteristic of expert nurses, although some were emphasized more than others.

Additional Competencies

Two domains — Organizational and Work Role Competencies and Monitoring and Ensuring the Quality of Health Care Practices — were expanded and new competencies were identified, reflecting the broader responsibilities in the system that are assumed by the master's prepared nurse. For example, one new area under Organization and Work Role Competencies was Competencies Developed to Cope with Staff Resistance to Change. Improving patient care through changes in the system was a frequent activity of the nurses in the sample, and they were highly skilled in determining the right timing and strategy to decrease resistance to change.

It was common to find these nurses doing extensive literature reviews before attempting to institute a change, so that they were able to speak to the opposition with documented research and clinical findings. One nurse described this as "bringing all her ammunition." Others were quite skillful in planning for change in advance and waiting for the most opportune time to introduce it.

Another example under the same domain was Making the Bureaucracy Respond to patients' and families' needs. The master's prepared nurses described a variety of creative ways of getting around the bureaucracy to meet those needs.

A new area which evolved in the domain of Monitoring and Ensuring the Quality of Health Care Practices was Recognition of a Generic Recurring Event or Problem That Requires a Policy Change. This skill involved the ability to discriminate between the idiosyncratic, isolated event that may jeopardize a patient's health and safety but is not likely to occur again and an event that also threatens a patient's health and safety and *is* likely to recur if policy changes are not made. This skill of identifying and evaluating recurring versus unique events effectively eliminates the situation that occurs in many bureaucratic settings where all patients are penalized inappropriately because one patient had a bad experience, for example, creating a restrictive policy about visiting, restraints, ambulation, or emergency procedures because a current policy was violated during an isolated incident.

A new domain, the Consulting Role of the Nurse, emerged out of the many examples given of the master's prepared nurses consistently providing expertise and guidance, both formally and informally, to other health care providers.

The results of our study documented that the master's prepared nurses in our sample possessed the competencies of expert nurses as identified by Benner. It

265

was also found that their roles were often broader and more complex than previously described in that they involved monitoring and evaluating care throughout the system.

In further analysis of the data, five categories emerged which have relevance for curriculum planning and evaluation. There were (1) dilemmas: ethical, clinical, and political; (2) positions or stances that breed success or failure; (3) nonarticulated common practices; (4) performance failures due to knowledge gaps; and (5) new knowledge, a blend of theoretical and empirical. Each category will be further described and its potential impact on curriculum planning and evaluation discussed.

Dilemmas

Many critical incidents presented dilemmas of one kind or another to the nurse and documented that the nurse is frequently required to make very painful and unpopular decisions. These critical incidents made lasting impressions on the nurses and have taken considerable time to resolve. Many of the ethical dilemmas that were presented involved prolonging life for the dying through artificial means and the policies related to resuscitation. It was obvious from the descriptions that the nurses seldom received assistance from physicians in resolving these dilemmas. Instead, their role was often to identify the issue and insist that the necessary decisions be made in a judicious way and by the responsible person.

Some dilemmas are both legal and political in nature. In one incident a nurse found herself in a clinic when a patient had a respiratory arrest. Both physicians present failed to act and told the nurse to find the physician who had ongoing knowledge of the patient. The master's prepared nurse resolved the issue by taking charge and responding appropriately. However, the incident points out the tremendous political and legal dilemmas faced by persons who take charge when both physicians and nurses are present at an emergency and the physicians fail to act or act inappropriately. Such situations raise many unanswered questions. In extreme emergencies such as this, formal role responsibilities and normal chains of commands shift to the person who is able to respond expertly in the situation at the moment.

It is clear from analysis of the incidents that most dilemmas result from the breakdown of clear-cut lines of authority when unpredictable emergency situations arise. The implication is that the successful nurse in a master's degree role should have specific skills not only to identify clinical, political, and ethical dilemmas but also to resolve the power and authority questions that contribute to the dilemmas. The implications for the curriculum are to determine if master's prepared nurses are being prepared adequately to identify the dilemmas and if they have the practical leadership training to identify the power and authority issues. Several successful strategies for dealing with the issues have been identified from these incidents and can now be included in the curriculum. The critical incidents provide excellent case studies for students to study and analyze as part of their clinical and core courses.

A Matter of Stances

Faculty has often questioned why some graduates are more successful in master's degree roles than others. The question is complex and not easily answered, because of all the immeasurable variables that go into successful performance. However, the data from this study identified some of the positions or stances taken by master's prepared nurses which appear to breed success or failure in their specific roles. Once identified, these positions or stances can be shared with graduate students so they can model or adopt the stances in their own practice.

A composite picture of successful nurses emerged from the collection of stances that breed success. One stance that seems to breed success is assertiveness with physicians with the expectation that the nurse is going to provide input into the situation. A successful master's prepared nurse will go to physicians' offices to discuss problems, attend their weekly conferences and programs, ask questions at grand rounds, and ask to present information at physician conferences. As one nurse said, "I think a lot of it has to do with suddenly realizing that it's just another person that you are talking to and you don't have to put them up on pedestals, so you're not intimidated by them and you feel more confident in what you're trying to present."

Other characteristics that lead to success are the development of an active support system; perserverance; the ability to listen to the concerns of others; knowing when to push for changes and when to wait; the ability to keep asking the right questions; and the ability to tolerate the ambiguities of the system. Each of these characteristics is illustrated by specific exemplars so that they can be more than context-free advice. For example, one nurse described her successful efforts in bringing about a major change in admission policy in order to individualize patient care and increase staff accountability. She related her willingness to meet and talk with other personnel, to listen to their concerns, and to persevere as the change took place slowly over a two-year period. Another nurse described her successful efforts in revising emergency policies for a clinic by choosing her time right after an emergency that pointed out the deficit dramatically to the department chairman and ensured his support.

Nonarticulated Practices

Common nonarticulated practices are those activities of the master's prepared nurse that are common to many situations but are usually not talked about, identified, or discussed. Counseling and supporting other nursing staff about low morale, burnout, and communication problems were commonly done but not indicated in formal job descriptions. Another behavior that was seen over and over was the guiding and coaching by the master's prepared nurse of other types of health care providers, including physicians, to help them to understand the patients' problems as the patients saw and experienced them.

More obvious was the nurses' relationship with their patients. The nurse–patient relationship was often observed and described as a warm, friendly, concerned, and positive attitude toward the patient. The nurses frequently touched their patients and sometimes hugged them during a very supportive and encouraging relationship. Often the nurse mentally placed herself in the role of the patient in order to recognize the indignities and traumas that patients often suffer at the hands of less sensitive health team members. Not only did the nurse recognize these indignities but she also pointed out the reality of the situation to other professionals and took steps to improve the situation, as the following example shows:

> *Nurse:* In the pediatric clinic it was common practice that the mother and child have to move from room to room to see each specialist, which might include several physicians, the social workers, and the dietician. I instituted a new plan whereby the mother and child would stay in the same room and the specialists would move from room to room. Several of the specialists said that they really didn't like the new system. They complained about having to carry their papers with them. I told them what it was like for the mother of a young child to move from room to room with the child, other siblings, a stroller, a diaper bag, a bottle, toys, and a purse and they finally understood why the change was necessary.

Other common practices were to break the rules when it is necessary for the patients' safety or care. In one example a nurse sent a pair of wire clippers home with a patient because her jaw was wired shut and she had to make a long airplane trip. Since the physician did not see the necessity of it, the nurse was unable to obtain them legitimately from the hospital so she just took them and had the patient mail them back after she arrived home. Another common practice is a real concern for what will happen to the patients after they return home. There were numerous examples of nurses making specific arrangements to insure that the home environment was supportive of a patient's convalescence and recovery.

Knowledge Gaps

Several knowledge gaps stands out. There are examples of difficulties in defining the role of the clinical specialist or master's-prepared nurse to other health professionals, such as physicians, social workers, and psychologists. This problem in defining the role of the nurse appears to cause nurses to have a diminished professional image and an inability to assess their real worth in the agency. Whether graduate programs fail to articulate the role or master's prepared nurses fail to define it is unclear. What is apparent, though, is that the master's prepared nurses in this sample reflected the use of concepts and principles taught in the program. They were able to demonstrate the role of the master's prepared nurse quite competently in both interviews and observations, but they often expressed their frustrations in articulating and justifying their worth to administrators and physicians.

Another knowledge gap seems to be understanding the different cultural and work values of other hospital personnel. The participants demonstrated a strong commitment to accepting and respecting different cultural values of the patients and families, but found it more difficult to work with the cultural differences of their coworkers, related to work expectations and values. It was as though they had learned to expect and communicate about cultural differences related to illness. However, typically, they were not prepared for the existing differences in work meanings and values of diverse coworkers.

New Knowledge

There were fewer examples of new knowledge, of an interaction of theoretical and empirical knowledge, but recognizing that this category exists has made us much more sensitive to those expert practices that may not yet be defined. In one example of how theoretical knowledge is applied in the clinical setting, a clinical specialist used Orem's theory of self-care as a way for nurses and team members from other disciplines to organize a plan of rehabilitation and independence for a severely disabled child. In this almost unbelievable example, the nurse persuaded the rehabilitation team to accept an eight-year-old child who was considered unable to be rehabilitated due to a lack of family support. The child had been severely burned and needed various prosthetic devices in order to do any self-care activities. She was neglected by her family and was not performing daily activities or going to school.

The nurse coordinated the team in teaching the child to be independent since she could not depend on her family; as the nurse stated, "It was a matter of survival." The child learned how to bathe and wash her hair, dress herself, and even cook her own meals even though she only had nubs for fingers and several prostheses. The final lesson was how to set her alarm so she could get up, dress herself, eat, and catch the school bus, all of which she eventually mastered. She returned to her family and was able to return to school. The incident reflected that the theory was applicable in even the most devastating of circumstances.

In another example a clinical specialist describes how she was able to tell the difference between exhaustion and postpartum psychosis in a new postpartum mother. She said:

I listened very carefully. A person who is exhausted has a certain way of speaking, but their logic is still there. They will deal with a question, they will hear you. A person who is psychotic will pick out something you have said and maybe halfway through the conversation come to the point. This person might say, but I love my baby, in the middle of a conversation that has to do with nipples. For example, I had asked are your nipples sore? And she responded: "But I love my baby." I would ask her questions that would show her ability to pick out what else was going on in her life. On the surface she might have appeared to someone else to be coping and answering appropriately until you really listened to the inappropriateness of it. Also I attend carefully to the way people look. This woman was sitting, hands together, leaning forward, staring at one spot, and taking her hand up to her hair and pushing it back. It's like she wanted to make herself into a ball.

This clinical specialist had been asked by the pediatrician to go into the home and make an assessment because he was uncertain about the parents' coping during an office visit. The clinical specialist made an accurate assessment of postpartum psychosis and arranged for the appropriate medical and psychiatric treatment.

Appraisal

This project is continuing and will include more data collection and analysis before conclusion. The final goal is to have a curriculum that is derived not only from theoretical knowledge but also from clinical knowledge from the practice setting. The faculty recognizes that after intensive study of these master's prepared nurses we have come up with more questions than answers. We believe, however, that the questions raised are the most relevant that a graduate nursing faculty could ask because they come from the issues, concerns, practice, and expertise of our graduates.

Although we are still a long way from our original goal, the improvement of the evaluation of the clinical component of the graduate program, we believe that what we have learned about the role of the master's prepared nurse is a first step that has contributed significantly to the development of our curriculum. The data and the interactions with the nurses in the study have given faculty a very realistic perception of the practice and work world of the master's prepared nurse. In the next year these data will be used to systematically evaluate the clinical components of the current curriculum to determine if and how they provide the basis for development of the competencies identified by the study.

The data will also be reviewed for sample case studies that faculty can use as examples of dilemmas faced by master's prepared nurses, along with successful and unsuccessful strategies used to resolve them. Knowledge gaps will be thoroughly studied, and additional instruction will be added to the curriculum where appropriate. The use of the critical incidents has already been integrated into several clinical courses as a way of focusing on expert practice and demonstrating the application of theory to practice.

There have been many unforeseen advantages of this approach to curriculum planning and evaluation. The faculty and master's prepared nurses in the hospital have worked closely together in the project, resulting in formal and informal sharing of ideas and collaborative efforts. Faculty have had opportunities to validate clincal practices with the nurses, and the nurses have been similary able to validate various education practices. It is the general perception of the faculty that the gap between practice and education has narrowed considerably since this project began and will continue to do so as it progresses.

Building Bridges Between Education and Practice

by *Kathleen Dolan, R.N., M.S.*
Assistant Director of Nursing Education and
Research, University of California, San Francisco

In the ten years since Kramer first described reality shock and its serious consequences to the nursing profession, numerous attempts have been made to bridge the gap between education and practice. A variety of pregraduation programs have been designed to introduce students to the work world values while they still remain in the protected environment of academia but are shortly to be launched into the realities of the practice setting. The number of articles describing special orientation programs for newly graduated nurses indicates that hospitals and health care agencies have also taken up the challenge of facilitating the transition of the neophyte nurse into the work setting. As a result, the senior student learns about reality shock while still in school and comes to the practice setting armed with helpful hints on becoming what Kramer (1974) calls bicultural. New nurses often examine themselves for symptoms of reality shock and can diagnose honeymoon phase behavior as easily as take vital signs.

Yet in spite of all these efforts, both neophyte and experienced nurses still find it difficult to base their practice on professional values. One new nurse recently described herself as a battleground on which school-bred values and practice values were in continuous skirmish, with shells and flak exchanged across no man's land. The battleground imagery reflects a pessimism in this young nurse, a pessimism stemming from a loss of hope in the eventual reconciliation of professional and bureaucratic values. New nurses want to make a difference in patient care, and those in nursing management want to coach them in ways that will enable them to maintain their idealism and vision while they are acquiring the skills and perspectives they need to become effective in the system.

The possibility of professional development after graduation and in the work setting that is offered by Benner's work with clinical knowledge acquisition can rekindle the hope of both neophyte and experienced nurses. The former can envision a progression from the advanced beginner stage to competency and beyond. The experienced nurse, whether competent, proficient, or expert, can gain insight into the unacknowledged domains of nursing practice and can learn to develop those areas openly and proudly.

At the University of California at San Francisco, nursing service has had a unique opportunity to collaborate with Benner in the application of the Dreyfus model and the clinical knowledge development framework to the practice setting. The close relationship between the school of nursing faculty and the University Hospitals nursing service personnel has facilitated cooperative program planning between Dr. Benner and the Division of Education and Research, the staff development arm of nursing service. The nurse educators in that division, excited by the potential for professional development in Benner's work, have incorporated some of the ideas and concepts derived from that work into the regular educational programming for staff employed at UCSF.

I Orientation Program

A lecture–discussion on the Dreyfus model and its application to nursing sets the tone for the first day of our orientation program for newly graduated nurses. Typically, these nurses have completed one month of hospital and unit orientation before the special program begins, during which time a staff nurse preceptor has been responsible for supervising their daily activities and monitoring progress.

A brief review of the AMICAE project establishes the disparity between perceptions of students, staff nurses, and nursing faculty as to the competencies of the new graduate. This is followed by a description of Benner's search for an explanation of this phenomenon through in-depth interviews with experienced nurses. Presentation of the Dreyfus model is followed by discussion of how this information can be useful in learning to function effectively in a new role. The neophyte learns that her proficient preceptor has the wisdom to know when a complicated dressing change should be done differently than the textbook suggests. The class hears, too, that the expert clinical nurse specialist operates on the basis of maxims that would be meaningless to the neophyte. The Dreyfus model offers the new nurses a framework for understanding the behavior of experienced nurses which, in the past, may have been interpreted through school-bred values as slipshod or mystical. They learn that *not* following a procedure is sometimes a matter of clinical judgment rather than a failure to meet standards of excellence.

Strategies for coping with a preceptor who forgets that the neophyte does not have the same perception of salience are discussed. The new nurse is encouraged to question the nurse specialist on the meanings of maxims. Through group discussion, these newly graduated nurses share recent experiences with competent, proficient, and expert nurses who illustrate the phases of the Dreyfus model. Lively debate often occurs as they attempt to determine whether their preceptors have attained proficiency or are merely competent. The most significant outcome of this session is the hope engendered in these neophyte nurses by this forward glimpse into a professional future, a future into which they can project their own development of clinical practice.

Preceptor Development

The staff nurse as preceptor for both the beginning and the experienced nurse is central to our orientation program. The preceptor is prepared through a day-long seminar that features the Dreyfus model as a key to understanding the behavior of new nurses, as a framework for appreciating the skill and knowledge gaps between preceptor and beginner, and as a basis for teaching strategies and evaluation methods.

Discussion of the model and the domains of nursing practice stimulates excitement among these competent, proficient, and expert nurses who are preparing to be preceptors. They readily recognize themselves in the descriptions of the stages in the model, nodding their heads and buzzing with their neighbors when reminded of what it was like not to have a sense of salience. Apart

from the direct impact this model has on their performance as preceptors, it clarifies for them the enormous
strides they have made in clinical knowledge development. They are encouraged to identify their current
clinical mastery and to consider their potential for future development.

Specific strategies for teaching the new nurse elicited
from Benner's work are discussed. Emphasis is placed
on using broad guidelines that help the advanced beginner deal with the particular demands of the unit, as well
as avoiding the use of maxims that go unexplained. The
preceptors are encouraged to maintain their practice
styles while monitoring themselves for divergence
from textbook solutions. Discussions with the preceptee at the end of the day focus on exploring the
context of the clinical situations that demand divergence. This balance between the broad guidelines and
the contextual allows the beginning nurse a degree of
comfort, since it uses a familiar learning style while
providing a glimpse of the perceptual grasp of the experienced nurse.

Although the focus of the presentation is on the neophyte nurse, the nurses in the preceptor development
course raise interesting questions about the applicability of the model to new employees who are
experienced nurses. Feeling a strong sense of responsibility to assist such nurses in learning the "UCSF way,"
the preceptors wonder whether the emphasis on hospital policies and procedures typical of an orientation
program will stifle the experienced nurse in building
clinical knowledge. The preceptors are encouraged to
project a sense of colleagueship with the experienced
nurse orientee, discussing different approaches to
clinical practice, exploring the context of a complex
clinical situation, and trading paradigm cases.

| Clinical Judgment Seminars

The existence of a well-developed clinical ladder at UCSF provides a unique opportunity for nurses of similar experiential background to meet and discuss their clinical practice, using Benner's work as the framework. Encouraged by the assistant director of nursing for surgery, a group of senior clinical nurses from several general surgical and surgical specialty units began a seminar series led by Benner to examine the context of their practice. In the initial session, Dr. Benner outlined the Dreyfus model and the domains of nursing practice and described the use of the critical incident technique to uncover the complexity and richness of nursing practice. Nurse educators from the staff development division came to learn the interpretive strategy used in group discussion.

Subsequent sessions focused on exploring and discussing the written critical incidents submitted in advance by the group members. The written descriptions invariably represented the bare facts of a situation, often without reference to the contextual material elicited by Benner through questioning and probing. The questions usually uncovered additional information about the patient as a person, the feelings the nurse had about the possibility for hope in the situation, and the goals she had for this particular patient.

As the sessions progressed, the participants shed the formal, often sterile language of a case presentation and adopted a more expressive style that described the context and reflected a strong holistic grasp of the situation. The incidents they presented moved from exciting emergency situations in which technology played a featured part to quieter, more patient-centered situations in which the use of self made the difference to a patient. The participants began to speak directly to each other as colleagues, acknowledging the contributions each had made to the patient situations.

The senior clinical nurses evaluated the seminar series as enriching to their professional practice and enhancing to each individual's sense of self as a nurse. One nurse commented that the seminars made her realize that when she had talked about "nursing," she had not really been talking about nursing practice. Evaluation by Dr. Benner and the nurse educators was accomplished by debriefing sessions after each seminar and after the series was completed. The concurrent debriefing sessions were essential for the nurse educators in learning the interpretive group technique.

The success of the clinical judgment seminar series in providing a forum for clinical nurses to discuss their practice and to uncover the knowledge embedded in that practice has stimulated the development of a monthly seminar for senior clinical nurses. Not yet fully implemented because of schedule constraints, the new series will follow the same format as described here and will be led by nurse educators trained by Dr. Benner.

Administrative Nurses

The administrative and managerial staff have been introduced to the Dreyfus model and to Benner's work through their regular monthly education programs. Prompted by Benner's speculation that the competent nurse may be a more appropriate choice as a preceptor for a new graduate than a proficient or expert nurse, the head nurses have encouraged their competent nurses to take the preceptor development course in preparation for assuming this role. The proficient and expert nurses are assigned as preceptors to the experienced new employees. Although no systematic evaluation has been done, informal responses indicate that the competent nurse preceptor who remembers what it was like to be a beginning nurse is sympathetic to the need for a formal, concrete approach to orientation.

All too aware of the beginning nurse's shortcomings, head nurses now have a framework for appreciating the potential that time and experience alone will unleash, given a challenging environment in which professional values are paramount. Several head nurses have altered the pace of their unit orientation programs in keeping with their understanding of the needs of the advanced beginner. Unfortunately, the needs of the more experienced nurse have been less well addressed, due in part to a failure to understand the nature of their needs plus the economic constraints and staffing demands to which head nurses must remain responsive. The head nurse may know quite clearly how to meet the needs of the experienced nurse for career development but be restrained by financial considerations.

| Summary

Driven by the burdens of staff turnover and the claims of changing technology, staff development departments have been forced to funnel precious resources away from programs that can be truly characterized as developmental and into programs that merely keep pace with changing personnel and more complex machines. Paradoxically, staff development departments often reinforce the staff nurse's contention that the acute care hospital is an inhospitable setting for career development. By responding only to the twin dragons of turnover and technology, staff development departments contribute unwittingly to the maintenance of an environment that does not advance professional practice. If career development assumed the same significance as new employee orientation and arrhythmia diagnosis in the educational programming of staff development departments, turnover and technology might be tamed, if not conquered.

The potential for career development that exists in Benner's work with the Dreyfus model is based on expanding our vision of the realities of nursing practice and knowledge. Staff development departments should provide a forum for discussion of clinical practice in which nursing knowledge is carefully charted and explored. Careful record keeping and sharing of paradigm cases are important strategies for documenting the significance of nursing practice. Teaching rounds by expert nurses open vistas to the advanced beginner and the competent nurse while recognizing the value of expertise and its importance in transmitting wisdom and judgment. Staff development departments have a significant role in creating the environment in which a new vision of nursing can be nurtured.

The many diverse and practical applications of this work are not easy to summarize. The most common finding is that nurses in different settings have looked at their practice and found wisdom and richness there that are not easily captured by formal models. We have a tradition of wanting only the best in nursing, and that is as it should be since we deal with life and death issues. Patients deserve the best, and we are aware that we want excellence for ourselves and our families when we need nursing care.

This zeal for excellence has sometimes made us attend only to the gaps and deficits. These five papers and the research reported in this book have demonstrated that we have much to learn from studying excellence. But, even more important, these studies illustrate that excellence and power are increasing, not deteriorating. After all, we cannot expect the recognition lag to disappear in society if it is still prevalent in nursing itself.

| References

Benner, P. May 1982. Issues in competency based testing. *Nursing Outlook 30*: (5), 303-309.

Benner, P. April 1983. Uncovering the knowledge embedded in clinical practice. *Image: The Journal of Nursing Scholarship.*

Benner, P. (1984) *Stress and satisfaction on the job: Work meanings and coping of mid-career men.* New York: Praeger.

Benner, P.; and Benner, R. 1979. *The new nurse's work entry: a troubled sponsorship.* New York: Tiresias Press.

Benner, P. et al. 1981. *From novice to expert: a community view of preparing for and rewording excellence in clinical nursing practice.* Unpublished report of the AMICAE Project (Grant No. 7 D10 29104-01), University of San Francisco.

Benner, P.; and Wrubel, J. May-June 1982. Clinical knowledge development: the value of perceptual awareness. *Nurse Educator 7*, 11-17.

Bellah, R. October 1982. Social science as practical reason. *The Hastings Center Report 12*(5), 32-39.

Berlew, D.E.; and Hall, T. 1964. *Some determinants of early managerial success.* Working Paper #81-64, Sloan School of Management, Massachusetts Institute of Technology, Cambridge, Mass.

Bourdieu, P. 1977. *Outline of a theory of practice.* Cambridge: Cambridge University Press.

Bracken, R.L.; and Christman, L. October 1978. An incentive program designed to develop and reward clinical competence. *Journal of Nursing Administration.*

Bray, D.W.; Campbell, R.J.; and Grant, D.L. 1974. *Formative years in business: a long-term AT&T study of managerial lives.* New York: John Wiley & Sons.

Breed, W. May 1955. Social control in the newsroom: a functional analysis. *Social Forces 133.*

Bursztajn, H. et al. 1981. *Medical choices, medical chances*. New York: Delacorte Press/Seymour Lawrence.

Carper, B.A. October 1978. Fundamental patterns of knowing in nursing. *Advances in Nursing Science 1*, 13-23.

Cassell, J. 1976. The contribution of social environment to host resistance. *American Journal of Epidemiology 104*, 107-33.

Colavecchio, R.; Tescher, B.; and Scalzi, C. October 1974. A clinical ladder for nursing practice. *Journal of Nursing Administration*.

Collins, R.N.; and Fielder, J.H. 1981. Becstrand's concept of practice theory: a critique. *Research in Nursing and Health 4*, 317-21.

Cousins, N. 1976. Anatomy of an illness (as perceived by the patient). *New England Journal of Medicine 295*, 1458-63.

Cousins, N. 1983. *The healing heart: antidotes to panic and helplessness*. New York: W.W. Norton.

Diers, D. November-December 1980. Nursing is a rich and confusing experience. *American Nurse 12*(4).

Dreyfus, H.L. 1979. *What computers can't do: the limits of artificial intelligence*. Revised ed. New York: Harper & Row.

Dreyfus, H.L. September 1980. Holism and hermeneutics. *Review of Metaphysics 34*, 3-23.

Dreyfus, H.L.; and Dreyfus, S.E. March 1977. *Uses and abuses of multi-attribute and multi-aspect model of decision making*. Unpublished manuscript, Department of Industrial Engineering and Operations Research, University of California at Berkeley.

Dreyfus, H.L.; and Dreyfus, S.E., with Athanasiou, T. (1986) *Mind over machine, the power of human intuition and expertise in the era of the computer*. New York: The Free Press.

Dreyfus, H.L.; and Rabinow, P. 1982. *Michael Foucault beyond structuralism and hermeneutics*. Chicago: University of Chicago Press, pp. xii-xxiii.

Dreyfus, S.E. 1982. Formal models vs. human situational understanding: inherent limitations on the modeling of business expertise. *Office: Technology and People 1*, 133-55.

Dreyfus, S.E.; and Dreyfus, H.L. February 1979. *The scope, limits, and training implications of three models of aircraft pilot emergency response behavior.* Unpublished report supported by the Air Force Office of Scientific Research (AFSC), USAF (Grant AFOSR-78-3594), University of California at Berkeley.

Dreyfus, S.E.; and Dreyfus, H.L. February 1980. *A five-stage model of the mental activities involved in directed skill acquisition.* Unpublished report supported by the Air Force Office of Scientific Research (AFSC), USAF (Contract F49620-79-C-0063), University of California at Berkeley.

Flanagan, M. *Summary of the public hearings.* July 1981. Chicago: National Commission on Nursing, American Hospital Association.

Gadamer, G. 1970. *Truth and method.* London: Sheer & Ward.

Geertz, C. 1973. *The interpretation of culture.* New York: Basic Books.

Gilligan, C. 1982. *In a different voice: psychological theory and women's development.* Cambridge: Harvard University Press.

Gilligan, C. 1983. Do the social sciences have an adequate theory of moral development? In N. Hann et al. (editors), *Social science as a moral inquiry.* New York: Columbia University Press.

Glaser, B.G. 1978. *Theoretical sensitivity.* Mill Valley, CA: Sociology Press.

Glaser, B.G.; and Strauss, A. 1967. *The discovery of grounded theory.* Chicago: Aldine.

Godfrey, M.A. 1978. Job satisfaction. *Nursing 78*, 8(4), 89-102.

Gordon, D.R. December 1981. *Geared toward change: hospital nursing's response to nursing turnover and nursing shortage.* Paper presented at the American

Anthropology Association Annual Meetings, Los Angeles, CA.

Gordon, D.R. December 1982. *A conflict between formal models of expertise and the development of expertise in American hospital nursing practice.* Paper presented at the American Anthropology Association Annual Meetings, Washington, DC.

Gordon, D.R. 1984. *Expertise, Formalism and Change in American Nursing Practice.* Doctoral dissertation, Medical Anthropology Program, University of California at San Francisco.

Greer, G. 1973. Woman power. In J.A. Ogilvy (editor), *Self and world: readings in philosophy.* New York: Harcourt Brace Jovanovich, pp. 410-12.

Hall, D.T.; and Hall, F.S. 1976. What's new in career management? *Organizational Dynamics* 5(1), 17-33.

Heidegger, M. 1962. *Being and time.* New York: Harper & Row.

Kesey, K. 1962. *One flew over the cuckoo's nest.* New York: Viking Press.

Kramer, M. 1974. *Reality shock: why nurses leave nursing.* St. Louis: C.V. Mosby.

Kramer, M.; and Baker, C. 1971. The exodus: can nursing afford it? *Journal of Nursing Administration* I(3), 15-30.

Kuhn, T.S. 1970. *The structure of scientific revolutions.* Chicago: University of Chicago Press.

Lazarus, R.S. 1985. The trivialization of distress. In Rosen, J.C., Solomon, I.J. (eds), *Preventing health risk behaviors and promoting coping with illness, Vol. 8 Vermont Conference on the Primary Prevention of Psychopathology.* Hanover, NH: University Press of New England.

Limon, S.; Spencer, J.; and Waters, V. May 1981. A clinical preceptorship to prepare reality-based ADN graduates. *Nursing and Health Care* 2(5), 267-69.

McClelland, D.C.; and Dailey, C. 1973. *Evaluating new methods of measuring the qualities needed in superior foreign service officers.* Boston: McBer.

Meintel, P.; and Rhodes, D.E. 1977. Clinical career ladder rewards RNs. *Hospital Progress.*

Menzies, I.E. 1960. A case study in the functioning of social systems as a defense against anxiety: a report of a study of the nursing service of a general hospital. *Human Relations* 13(2), 101-9.

Neill, S.B. 1978. *The competency movement: problems and solutions.* Washington, DC: American Association of School Administrators, Critical Issues Report.

Palmer, R.E. 1969. *Hermeneutics.* Evanston, IL: Northwestern University Press.

Polanyi, M. 1958. *Personal Knowledge.* London: Routledge & Kegan Paul.

Pottinger, P. 1975. *Comments and guidelines for research in competency identification, definition and measurement.* Report prepared for the Educational Policy Research Center, Syracuse University (ERIC document ED134541).

Rabinow, P.; and Sullivan, M. 1979. *Interpretive social science.* Berkeley: University of California Press.

Sandel, M. 1982. *Liberalism and the limits of justice.* London: Oxford University Press.

Schein, E.H. 1968. Organizational socialization and the profession of management. *Industrial Management Review* 9, 1-16.

Selye, H. 1969. *Stress without distress.* New York: McGraw-Hill Book Company.

Skipper, J.K., Jr. 1965. The role of the hospital nurse: Is it instrumental or expressive? In J.K. Skipper, Jr.,; and R.C. Leonard (editors), *Social interaction and patient care.* Philadelphia: J.B. Lippincott, pp. 40-48.

Steinbeck, J. 1941. The Mexican Sierra. In *The log from the sea of Cortez.* New York: Viking. Quoted in K. Weick, 1979. *Social psychology of organizing.* 2nd ed. Reading, MA: Addison-Wesley, p. 29.

Stotland, E. 1969. *The psychology of hope.* San Francisco: Jossey-Bass.

Sudnow, D. 1978. *Ways of the hand: the organization of improvised conduct.* Cambridge: Harvard University Press.

Tanner, C.A. 1983. Research on clinical judgment. In W. Holzemer (editor), *Review of research in nursing education*. New Jersey: Slack Publishers, pp. 1-32.

Taylor, C. September 1971. Interpretation and the sciences of man. *The Review of Metaphysics 25*(1), 3-34, 45-51.

Taylor, C. 1982. Dawes Hicks lecture. Theories of meaning. Paper read November 6, 1980, *Proceedings of the British Academy*, pp. 283-327.

Thomas, L. 1983. *The youngest science: notes of a medcine-watcher*. New York: Viking Press.

Walton, R.E. 1974. Innovative restructuring of work. In J. Rosow (editor), *The worker and the job: coping with change*. Englewood Cliffs, NJ: Prentice-Hall, pp. 145-76.

Walton, R.E. 1975. Improving the quality of work-life. Harvard Business Review on Management. San Francisco: Harper & Row.

Weed, L.L. 1970. *Medical records, medical education, and patient care*. Chicago: Year Book Medical Publishers.

Wilson, H.S. 1977. Limiting intrusion—social control of outsiders in a healing community. *Nursing Research 26*(2), 103-10.

Wrubel, J.: Benner, P.; and Lazarus, R.S. 1981. Social competence from the perspective of stress and coping. In J.D. Wine and M.D. Smye (editors), *Social competence*. New York: Guilford Press, pp. 61-99.

Yankelovich, D. 1974. The meaning of work. In J. Rosow (editor), *The worker and the job: coping with change*. Englewood Cliffs, NJ: Prentice-Hall.

Glossary

Advanced beginner   A stage in the Dreyfus model. One who can demonstrate marginally acceptable performance; one who has coped with enough real situations to note, or to have pointed out by a mentor, recurring meaningful situational components. The *advanced beginner* has enough background experience to recognize aspects of a situation.

Aspects of a situation   Cannot be described in a context-free way; can be understood only by a person with prior experience or understanding of the situation. For example, recognizing a patient's readiness to learn or recognizing signs of withdrawal in children (due to depression over being separated from their parents) require prior experience with these concrete situations before they can be reliably recognized. *Aspects of a situation* can never attain the degree of certainty or clarity that is possible with attributes or measurable properties.

Attributes of a situation   Quantifiable features or properties that can be adequately explained without prior exposure to a real situation. For example, the nurse can learn to take temperature or blood pressure readings without prior knowledge of situations where blood pressure or temperatures are measured.

Clinical knowledge development   Examination and description of practical knowledge or know-how gained from clinical experience. Clinical knowledge is embedded in expert practice and can be discovered or "uncovered" by interpretive and ethnographic studies in actual clinical settings.

Competency   An interpretively defined area of skilled performance identified and described by its intent, function, and meanings (as in *competency* statement). This use of *competency* is unrelated to the competent stage in the Dreyfus Model of Skill Acquisition (see below).

Competent   A stage in the Dreyfus model of skill acquisition typified by considerable conscious, deliberate planning. The plan dictates which attributes and aspects of the current and contemplated future situation are to be considered most important and which can be ignored. The *competent* stage is evidenced by an increased level of efficiency.

Common meanings   Taken-for-granted or background knowledge that is not socially negotiated in an explicit way. *Common meanings* make it possible for persons to communicate directly and understand one another without interpretation or translation. People who share a common culture and language have a background of common meanings. Subcultures such as disciplinary groups (work groups) develop common meanings that become embedded in their work practices and expectations.

Descriptive rules Explanatory statements that descriptively account for regularity in behaviors. An ethnographer or linguist might develop *descriptive rules* to account for regularities in pauses in speech or in distance-standing behaviors. However, neither would claim that these *descriptive rules* are "unconscious" generative rules being followed by the participants; in other words, the behaviors are not generated by the rules.

Dreyfus model of skill acquisition Developed by Stuart E. Dreyfus and Hubert L. Dreyfus, both professors at the University of California at Berkeley. This is a situational model of skill acquisition, as opposed to a trait or talent model. Since this model is situational, performance level can be determined only by consensual validation of expert judges and assessment of the outcomes of a situation. Reliability is determined by inter-rater agreement between experts by repeated assessments. This model was originally developed in a study of chess players and pilots and was extended to nursing practice in a field study.

Domain A *domain* of practice is a cluster of competencies that have similar intents, functions, and meanings.

Exemplar Refers to an example that conveys more than one intent, meaning function or outcome and can easily be compared or translated to other clinical situations whose objective characteristics might be quite different. An *exemplar* might be a paradigm case for a clinician. Kuhn (1970) used the word *exemplar* for scientific experiments that guide subsequent scientific works. The term has a more heuristic import and conveys a more active stance than a specific example or instance.

Experience Transactions count as *experience* only when the person actively refines preconceived notions and expectations. This "negative" view of *experience* has positive outcomes. Experience is gained when theoretical knowledge is refined, challenged, or disconfirmed by actual clinical evidence that enhances or runs counter to the theoretical understanding.

Expertise Developed only when the clinician tests and refines theoretical and practical knowledge in actual clinical situations. *Expertise* develops through a process of comparing whole similar and dissimilar clinical situations with one another, so an expert has a deep background understanding of clinical situations based upon many past paradigm cases. *Expertise* is a hybrid of practical and theoretical knowledge.

Formal model A theoretical scheme of patterns of causality, interactions, and relationships. A *formal model* is based upon practical knowledge of the real world. It is a simplified view or scheme of the situation that captures what is considered the most influential factors of the situation. *Formal models* are useful for orienting beginners to a situation, so they will ask fruitful questions and attend to important resources, constraints, and demands in the situation.

Generative rules Rules that create behavior. The stance taken in this book is that there are no *generative rules* or deep structures, laws or mechanisms that generate behavior in a mechanistic, interpretation-free way.

Graded qualitative distinctions Distinctions dependent upon human perceptual abilities and not reducible to context-free or elemental quantitative measurements. *Graded qualitative distinctions* require expert human recognitional abilities similar to those acquired by a connoisseur. Tonicity of the premature infant, degree of cyanosis, or respiratory distress are examples of graded qualitative distinctions.

Informal models Situational, context-dependent human knowledge based upon prior experience. *Informal models* consist of whole concrete past experiences that have become exemplars or paradigm cases. *Informal models* rely on skills and human relationships, not just symbolic or formal knowledge.

Intuitive grasp Direct apprehension of a situation based upon a background of similar and dissimilar situations and embodied intelligence or skill. *Intuitive grasp* is never "blind" as is a wild guess, but relies on perceptual capacity based upon prior experience. *Intuitive grasp* should not be confused with mysticism, since it is available only in situations where a deep background understanding of the situation exists, based upon a broad base of knowledge and experience. *Intuitive grasp* makes expert human decision making possible. It allows a gestalt or holistic understanding that bypasses building the situation up element by element and then grouping or synthesizing the elements into a conclusion or whole picture. *Intuitive grasp* is not possible without a sufficient background and experience with many similar and dissimilar situations.

Knowledge utilization The application of theories and knowledge gained from research and the latest scientific and technological discoveries in the clinical setting.

Maxim   A cryptic description of skilled performance that can benefit one who has enough skill to recognize the implications of the instructions. For example, a *maxim* in sports would be a phrase like "keep your eye on the ball," which means little to the beginner but is applicable to the skilled player. Experts exchange *maxims* in clinical practice: "There's a difference between 'working in the grey zone,' 'chasing the problem,' and 'aggressively chasing the problem'." These distinctions vary (given the patient population) and require a certain level of expertise for interpretation.

Novice   That stage in the Dreyfus model of skill acquisition where no background understanding of the situation exists, so that context-free rules and attributes are required for safe entry and performance in the situation. It is *unusual* for a graduate nurse to be a *novice*, but it is possible. For example, an expert nurse in gerontology would be a *novice* in a neonatal intensive care unit. Many first-year nursing students will begin at the novice stage; however, students who have had experience as nurse's assistants will *not* be *novice* in basic nursing skills. In this book, *novice* should *not* be attributed to the newly graduated nurse because, in most cases, the newly graduated nurse will perform at the advanced-beginner level.

Paradigm case   A clinical episode that alters one's way of understanding and perceiving future clinical situations. These cases stand out in the clinician's mind; they are reference points in their current clinical practice. *Paradigm cases* form the bases for predictions and projections. They can easily be communicated if the lesson is simple (describing how an error might occur or be prevented), but if the knowledge is more complex and dependent upon many other *paradigm cases* or personal knowledge, it cannot be translated to another clinician, unless the other clinician has a similar fund of personal knowledge and *paradigm cases. Paradigm cases* are exemplars that become a part of the clinician's perceptual lens.

Practical knowledge   Knowledge gained through directly practicing skills and taking up cultural practices. It is "knowing how" as opposed to "knowing that." Many skills are acquired without formal explanations to explain why the skill is possible, or without the formal laws to capture the principles that make the skill feasible. Bicycle riding and swimming are two common skills that do not yet have satisfactory formal explanations.

Proficient   A stage in the Dreyfus model. The *proficient* performer perceives situations as wholes rather than in terms of aspects, and performance is guided by maxims. There is a qualitative leap or discontinuity in problem approach between the *proficient* and the competent level of performance. The *proficient* performer recognizes a situation in terms of the overall picture. This person recognizes which aspects of the situation are *most* salient. The *proficient* performer has an intuitive grasp of the situation based upon a deep background understanding.

Rule-governed behavior   Behavior that is inflexible because it attends only to what can be stated explicitly in rules. *Rule-governed behavior* ignores the nuances and exceptions in a situation. So instead of rules being guidelines or statements of minimal expectations or standards, they become restrictive when applied in a literal, legalistic way. The very intent and spirit of a rule can be violated in *rule-governed behavior*.

Salience   The condition where certain aspects stand out as more or less important in a situation. *Salience* is a perceptual stance or embodied knowledge whereby a person does not deliberately have to calculate which aspects of the situation are more or less important; they just *appear* as more or less important. People with a sense of *salience* selectively ignore the less important aspects of the situation (from their learned perspective) and are sensitive to nuances that might influence the more significant aspects. This view of *salience* is not dependent upon a representational view of knowledge but rather asserts that the knower (unlike a computer) has direct access to the situation through skills, and a committed stance. For the expert, what is *salient* will be taken for granted, as "just the way the world is" or as obvious. However, if the expert is to maintain or extend his or her expertise, that which is salient will necessarily be challenged and will therefore shift as a result of new information and experience.

Theoretical knowledge   A formal statement of the necessary and sufficient conditions for the occurrence of real situations. *Theoretical knowledge* is "knowing that" and includes formal statements about interactional and causal relationships between events.

| Appendix

| Guideline for Recording Critical Incidents

Developed by
Deborah R. Gordon and Patricia Benner

The AMICAE Project
University of San Francisco
2130 Fulton, San Francisco, CA 94117

You have been asked by the AMICAE Project staff to describe critical incidents from your clinical practice. These incidents will serve as a basis for developing competency-based exams for follow-through evaluation of new graduates for the local schools of nursing. They will also be used as the baseline material for a publication on the nature of applied nursing practice, with particular focus on the significance of experience in clinical practice in differentiation of the novice and experienced clinician.

The attached forms can be used to record your critical incident. First, however, some clarification of what is meant by critical incident is in order. It includes *any* of the following types of incidents.

A. What Constitutes a Critical Incident

- An incident in which you feel your intervention really made a difference in patient outcome, either directly or indirectly (by helping other staff members)
- An incident that went unusually well
- An incident in which there was a breakdown (i.e., things did not go as planned)
- An incident that is very ordinary and typical
- An incident that you think captures the quintessence of what nursing is all about
- An incident that was particularly demanding

*Spacing in this questionnaire has been condensed for publication in this book.

B. What to Include in Your Description of a Critical Incident

- The context of the incident (e.g., shift, time of day, staff resources)
- A detailed description of what happened
- Why the incident is "critical" to you
- What your concerns were at the time
- What you were thinking about as it was taking place
- What you were feeling during and after the incident
- What, if anything, you found most demanding about the situation

C. Personal Data

Name: (optional)   Date:
Title:
Institution:
Amount of time on current unit:
Amount of time in nursing practice:
Unit where incident took place:

D. In the space below, please describe in detail a critical incident from your nursing practice, addressing the questions outlined in Part B.

E. Please use the space below to describe a critical incident from your nursing practice in which you recently participated.

1. In what way was this incident critical?
2. What were your concerns at the time?
3. What were you thinking about as it was taking place?
4. What were your feelings during and after the incident?
5. What, if anything, did you find particularly demanding about the incident?
6. What did you find particularly satisfying about the incident?

F. A Typical Day at Work

In the space below, please describe to us a typical day you have had recently at your work.

G. An Unusual Day at Work

In the space below, please describe a day at your work that was unusual in some significant way.

In the past, we have found it very helpful to collect accounts of the same incident from more than one participant, particularly participants who differ in the amount of experience they have had in clinical nursing practice. We thus would welcome any further accounts of this incident by other staff members who were involved in what took place. We would also welcome any comments or questions you might have.

Index

303